Brain Diet Recipes

For

Seniors

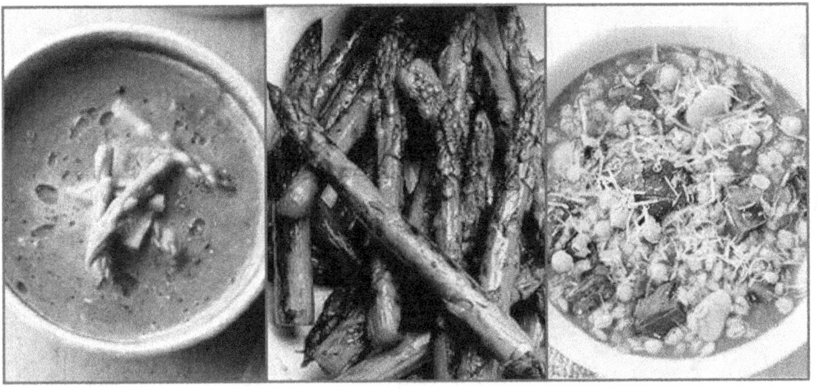

Nurturing Aging Cognitive Function Through Food

Mary J. Abbey

Table of Content

INTRODUCTION

Emily was an old woman who lived in a little town, she was a lovely and compassionate woman, but lately, she had been feeling forgetful more and more. She frequently forgot appointments or her keys, and she was beginning to worry that she was getting dementia.

Emily once stumbled upon a cookbook with brain diet recipes when she was at the library. She curiously picked it up, and the more she read, the more certain she was that she had to give it a try.

According to the book, several meals are especially beneficial for enhancing brain function. Foods like fish, almonds, berries, and leafy green vegetables are among these. Recipes for a variety of meals and snacks that might sharpen the mind were also included in the book.

Emily chose to experiment with the brain diet. She started by consuming more of the suggested meals and started preparing some of the recipes in the book. She was pleasantly pleased by how good the food was, and she noticed that after eating, she felt more focused and attentive.

Emily's memory significantly improved after a few weeks on the brain diet. She could now carry on conversations more fluidly and stopped misplacing her keys or forgetting appointments. She decided to go with the brain diet permanently since she was so pleased with the outcomes.

Emily once informed Susan, a friend of hers, about the brain diet. Susan, who was likewise elderly, had been having similar issues with her memory. Susan was persuaded to try the brain diet by Emily, and Susan was astounded by the results.

As regular cooking partners, Emily and Susan frequently tried out novel dishes that were thought to be beneficial for the brain. Additionally, they would spread the word about their meals to other friends and family members, and before long, the brain diet was the talk of the town.

Emily and her friends' memory and cognitive performance were enhanced as a result of the brain diet. They were all happier and more interested in life, and they were appreciative of the second chance the brain diet had provided for them.

CHAPTER ONE

Connection Between Food and Brain Healthy

In essence, the relationship between food and brain health is profound. The nutrients we consume directly impact the structure and functioning of our brain. Omega-3 fatty acids found in fish, flaxseeds, and walnuts, for instance, support cognitive function and can aid in reducing the risk of cognitive decline.

Antioxidants from fruits and vegetables, like berries and spinach, help combat oxidative stress, which is linked to brain aging and neurodegenerative diseases. B vitamins, present in whole grains and leafy greens, contribute to the production of neurotransmitters, vital for mood regulation and cognitive processes.

Moreover, a balanced diet maintains stable blood sugar levels, fostering optimal brain activity. Foods with a low glycemic index, such as whole grains and lean proteins, prevent energy crashes and aid concentration.

Gut health also influences brain health. Probiotic-rich foods like yogurt can positively affect gut bacteria, potentially benefiting mental well-being through the gut-brain axis.

Conversely, diets high in saturated fats and refined sugars may impair cognitive function and promote inflammation, potentially increasing the risk of conditions like dementia and depression.

In summation, a diet rich in nutrient-dense foods - encompassing a variety of fruits, vegetables, lean proteins, healthy fats, and whole grains - can significantly contribute to maintaining and enhancing brain health throughout life.

Nutrients Essential for Cognitive Function

The cognitive processes of learning, memory, attention, problem-solving, and attentiveness play a significant role in our daily lives. Proper diet has a significant impact on cognitive health because certain nutrients support good brain function and mental well-being in general.

It's crucial to keep up a balanced diet full of these essential nutrients to enhance cognitive function and mental health. It's critical to keep in mind, however, that factors associated with a healthy lifestyle as a whole, such as regular exercise, adequate sleep, and mental stimulation, are also very important for preserving cognitive function throughout time.

CHAPTER TWO

Building a Brain-Boosting Foundation

Strengthening our cognitive talents is important if we want to live happy and rewarding lives. To improve our ability to learn, solve problems, and perform other cognitive tasks, it is important to lay a foundation for brain health.

The following are the key principles to consider in this journey:

Healthy Lifestyle: A sound body is the basis for a strong intellect. To function at its best, the brain needs regular exercise, a well-balanced diet full of nutrients, and enough sleep. While healthy eating supplies the required energy for cognitive activities, physical activity promotes blood flow to the brain

Mindful Mental Stimulation: Just as physical exercise strengthens muscles; mental exercises stimulate the brain. Engaging in activities such as puzzles, brainteasers, reading, and learning new skills keeps the brain active and adaptable. Continuous learning fosters neuroplasticity, allowing the brain to reorganize and form new connections.

Social Engagement: Human interaction plays a pivotal role in cognitive health. Engaging in conversations, participating in social activities, and maintaining meaningful relationships provide cognitive challenges and emotional support that contribute to mental well-being.

Stress Management: The brain might suffer harm from prolonged stress. Practicing stress management techniques like mindfulness, meditation, and relaxation exercises can help reduce stress hormone levels, supporting better cognitive function.

Quality Sleep: Sleep is when the brain consolidates memories and performs essential maintenance. Prioritize getting 7-9 hours of quality sleep each night to support cognitive restoration and overall brain health.

Balanced Mental Workload: Striking a balance between mental challenges and relaxation is crucial. While pushing your cognitive limits is important, it's equally essential to give your brain periods of rest to prevent burnout.

Continual Curiosity: Cultivate a curious mindset that seeks to explore, question, and learn novelty, and stepping out of your comfort zone stimulates brain activity and encourages creative thinking.

Brain-Boosting Foods: Certain foods, such as fatty fish rich in omega-3 fatty acids, berries loaded with antioxidants, and nuts abundant in healthy fats, are believed to support brain health. Incorporating these into your diet can provide a nutritional boost to your cognitive foundation.

Stay Hydrated: Proper hydration is vital for optimal brain function. Dehydration can impair concentration and cognitive abilities, so remember to drink enough water throughout the day.

Positive Outlook: Maintaining a positive attitude and managing negative emotions effectively can contribute to cognitive resilience. Positive emotions have been linked to improved problem-solving skills and enhanced overall cognitive performance.

Remember that building a brain-boosting foundation is a lifelong tot requires consistent effort and commitment. By integrating these principles into your daily life, you can pave the way for a sharper, more resilient mind that supports your personal and professional growth.

Understanding the Aging Brain

Given its substantial effects on human cognition and well-being, the study of the aging brain has attracted a lot of attention in the field of neuroscience. Memory, attention, and problem-solving skills are just a few of the cognitive capabilities that can be affected by the complex series of changes the brain goes through as we age. This note briefly explores several significant discoveries about the aging brain.

First, the aging brain undergoes structural changes. The size of the brain tends to decrease, and some areas like the prefrontal cortex, which controls executive functions experience more significant decreases. As we get older, these changes may make multitasking, making decisions, and planning more difficult.

Second, adjustments are made to neuronal connections. Other compensatory connections can emerge as certain connections deteriorate or weaken, making it more difficult to process information. This phenomenon may assist in explaining why older people may develop techniques to slow cognitive aging, using different parts of the brain for different tasks.

Thirdly, aging brain research has memory changes as a main focus. While long-term memory typically remains stable or even improves, short-term memory may start to become less trustworthy. When compared to semantic memory, which deals with broad knowledge, episodic memory, which involves personal events, may see higher reductions.

Fourthly, the environment, lifestyle, and heredity all have a significant impact on how the aging brain develops. Maintaining cognitive vigor in later years is linked to regular physical activity, a healthy diet, mental stimulation, and social interaction.

Importance of Proactive Brain Care

In essence, cultivating our brain's health is as important as maintaining our physical health. Proactively caring for our brains enables us to excel in both our personal and professional endeavors while also improving our general quality of life. After all, a healthy brain serves as the foundation for both an individual's happiness and a prosperous society.

A variety of tactics are used in proactive brain care to improve cognitive resilience and avert prospective problems. The cornerstone of such care is regular exercise, a balanced diet full of nutrients that support brain function, and adequate rest. Mental agility is enhanced by intellectual challenges and unique experiences because they stimulate brain pathways.

Proactive brain care also includes stress reduction methods like mindfulness and meditation. Chronic stress can alter the anatomical makeup of the brain in addition to impairing cognitive function. People can maintain their brain's health and function by reducing stress.

As we become older, putting brain health first becomes more important. Although age-related cognitive decline is a fact, its commencement can be postponed by taking preventive steps. Learning a new skill or language is an example of an activity that promotes neuroplasticity and can create new connections between neurons while protecting the brain from deterioration.

Overuse of screens and information overload can tax cognitive resources in the digital era. Setting limits on screen time and allotting time for mental rest and renewal are both components of proactive brain care.

CHAPTER THREE

Keys Nutrients for Brain Health

1. Omega-3 Fatty Acids: Found in fatty fish like salmon, walnuts, and flaxseeds, omega-3 fatty acids are essential for brain health. They contribute to the structural integrity of brain cells and aid in the transmission of signals between neurons, which is vital for memory and cognitive processing.

2. Antioxidants (Vitamins C and E): Vitamins C and E, abundant in fruits, vegetables, nuts, and seeds, act as powerful antioxidants. They protect brain cells from oxidative stress and inflammation, which can contribute to cognitive decline over time.

3. B Vitamins: B vitamins, especially B6, B9 (folate), and B12, are involved in producing neurotransmitters that regulate mood and cognitive function. They can be found in foods like leafy greens, eggs, lean meats, and whole grains.

4. Magnesium: Magnesium, present in nuts, seeds, whole grains, and leafy greens, is essential for synaptic plasticity the brain's ability to adapt and change, crucial for learning and memory.

5. Choline: Choline, found in eggs, liver, and certain vegetables, supports neurotransmitter synthesis and plays a role in memory and learning.

6. Vitamin D: Apart from its role in bone health, vitamin D is also linked to cognitive function. Exposure to sunshine and fortified meals like dairy products can both provide it.

7. Iron: Iron, present in red meat, beans, and fortified cereals, supports oxygen transport to brain cells. Fatigue and reduced cognitive function are two effects of iron insufficiency.

8. Zinc: Zinc, found in foods like meat, nuts, and legumes, plays a role in neurotransmitter function and overall cognitive development.

9. Protein: Amino acids from dietary protein sources are crucial for neurotransmitter production, which influences mood and cognitive performance.

10. Polyphenols: These plant compounds, abundant in berries, dark chocolate, tea, and some vegetables, have antioxidant and anti-inflammatory properties that support cognitive health.

Omega-3 Fatty Acids: Fuel for Thought

Omega-3 fatty acids: little molecules have a huge effect. These vital fats are not only needed for sustaining general health but also serve a significant role in nourishing the brain, our body's most complex organ. Omega-3s, often known as "Fuel for Thought," are a crucial dietary element that enhances mental acuity, memory, and emotional health.

The recommended nutrients for the brain are DHA (docosahexaenoic acid) and EPA (eicosapentaenoic acid), two forms of omega-3s found in fatty fish like salmon, mackerel, and sardines. The structural integrity of brain cells is built and maintained by these fatty acids, according to research, which promotes effective neuronal communication. As a result, they support greater cognitive capacities like better problem-solving, crystal-clear thinking, and focus.

Omega-3 fatty acids also have anti-inflammatory effects in addition to improving cognitive function. Numerous neurodegenerative disorders, such as Alzheimer's disease and Parkinson's disease, have been related to contortion in the brain. Omega-3s may potentially lower the risk of various illnesses by reducing inflammation, hence long-term boosting brain health.

Notably, the benefits of omega-3 fatty acids don't just apply to adults; they also have an impact on fetal development. DHA, a significant omega-3 component, is essential for prenatal brain development. Pregnant women who include omega-3-rich items in their diets may help their offspring develop cognitively and emotionally.

Antioxidants: When the body's free radicals and antioxidants are in an unbalanced ratio, oxidative stress results. Free radicals are unstable molecules generated as a byproduct of normal bodily processes, such as metabolism, or due to external factors like pollution and UV radiation. Cells, proteins, and DNA can become damaged when the number of free radicals exceeds the number of antioxidants. This damage has been linked to a range of health problems, including aging, cardiovascular diseases, cancer, and neurodegenerative disorders.

Antioxidants, found in various fruits, vegetables, nuts, and whole grains, act as powerful defenders against this damage. They neutralize free radicals by donating electrons, effectively breaking the chain reaction of cell destruction. Common antioxidants include vitamins such as vitamin C, vitamin E, and beta-carotene, as well as minerals like selenium and zinc. Flavonoids, polyphenols, and other phytochemicals present in plant-based foods also exhibit antioxidant properties.

Regular consumption of antioxidant-rich foods is essential to maintain a balance between free radicals and antioxidants. These foods include berries, citrus fruits, leafy greens, nuts, and colorful vegetables. Additionally, a healthy lifestyle that includes regular exercise, stress management, and sufficient sleep supports the body's antioxidant defense mechanisms.

Research suggests that antioxidants offer more than just protection against oxidative stress. They may play a role in reducing inflammation, supporting immune function, and even promoting healthy skin. However, it's important to note that the benefits of antioxidants are best realized when obtained through a balanced diet rather than relying solely on supplements.

Vitamins and Minerals: Nourishing Cognitive Function

Vitamins such as B-complex vitamins (B6, B9, B12), vitamin D, and vitamin E are known for their cognitive benefits. B-complex vitamins are involved in the synthesis of neurotransmitters, the chemical messengers that enable communication between brain cells. Vitamin D supports brain health by promoting nerve growth, reducing inflammation, and regulating calcium levels crucial for neuron communication. Vitamin E, a powerful antioxidant, helps protect brain cells from oxidative stress, which can lead to cognitive decline.

Minerals like iron, zinc, magnesium, and iodine also contribute to cognitive well-being. Iron is vital for delivering oxygen to the brain, ensuring proper energy production. Zinc supports neurotransmitter function and assists in forming new neural connections. Magnesium plays a role in synaptic plasticity, the brain's ability to adapt and learn. Iodine, essential for thyroid function, indirectly impacts cognitive development, especially during infancy and childhood.

A balanced diet rich in fruits, vegetables, whole grains, lean proteins, and healthy fats provides the necessary vitamins and minerals to support cognitive function. As we age, maintaining these nutrient levels becomes increasingly important to prevent cognitive decline and promote brain health.

CHAPTER FOUR

Brain Boosters Recipes and Preparation

The brain is one of the most essential organs in the body, and it needs the correct nutrition to work at its optimum. A balanced diet can help enhance brain function, memory, and cognitive decline.

In our fast-paced lives, it's crucial to nourish our brains with the right nutrients to maintain mental clarity, focus, and memory. Incorporating these recipes and meal plans into your routine can be a delicious and rewarding way to support your brain health.

The Brain Booster Diet is a strategy of eating that concentrates on foods that are excellent for the brain. Crafting a brain-healthy meal plan involves incorporating a variety of nutrient-dense foods that nourish both the body and mind. Remember to include omega-3 fatty acids, antioxidants, vitamins and minerals, whole grains, lean proteins, healthy fats, and a rainbow of fruits and vegetables to provide a comprehensive range of essential nutrients to promote brain health.

Salsa spaghetti with sardines

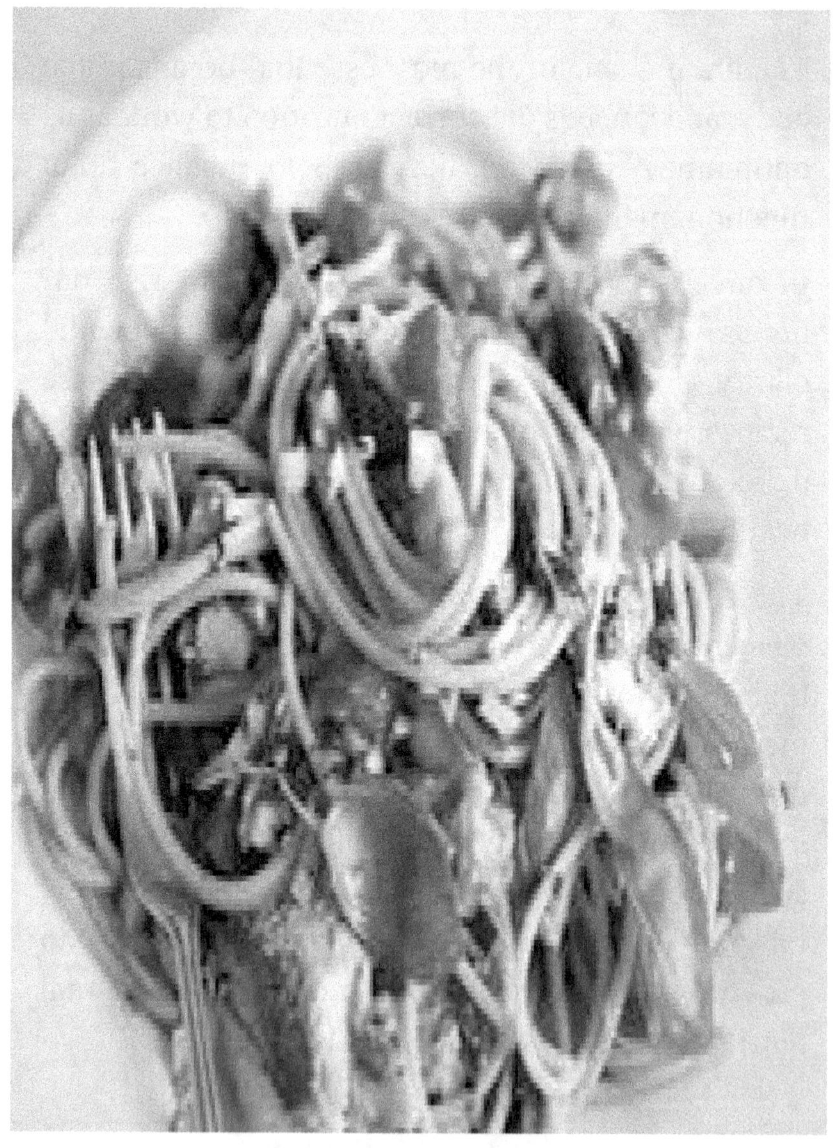

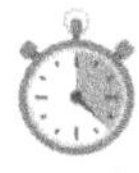

Prep time= 15 minutes

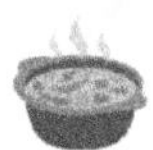

Cooking time= 15 minutes

INGREDIENTS

100 grams of whole-wheat spaghetti
2 large, ripe tomatoes, cut finely
One red onion, very finely chopped, fifteen pitted black Kalamata olives, quartered, and one-half teaspoon of red chili juice and zest, also finely chopped. 12 lemons, as desired

1 teaspoon of fresh oregano or 4 tablespoons of basil, chopped

Sardines in olive oil, two 120g cans, emptied with oil saved

Nutrient Unit

Kcal: 440
Fat: 15.8g
Saturates 2.9g
Carbs: 42.9g
Sugars: 9.5g
Fiber: 6.9g
Protein: 29.5g
low in salt: 1.6g

INSTRUCTION

STEP 1
Boil the spaghetti according to the directions on the package. Combine the tomatoes, onion, olives, chili, lemon zest, and basil or oregano while you wait. Sardines can be heated in a pan or a microwave.
STEP 2
Drain the pasta and add it back to the pan with the tomato mixture. Toss well. Add the chunky bits of sardines. If desired, season with pepper, lemon juice, and some canning oil.

Basque-style salmon stew

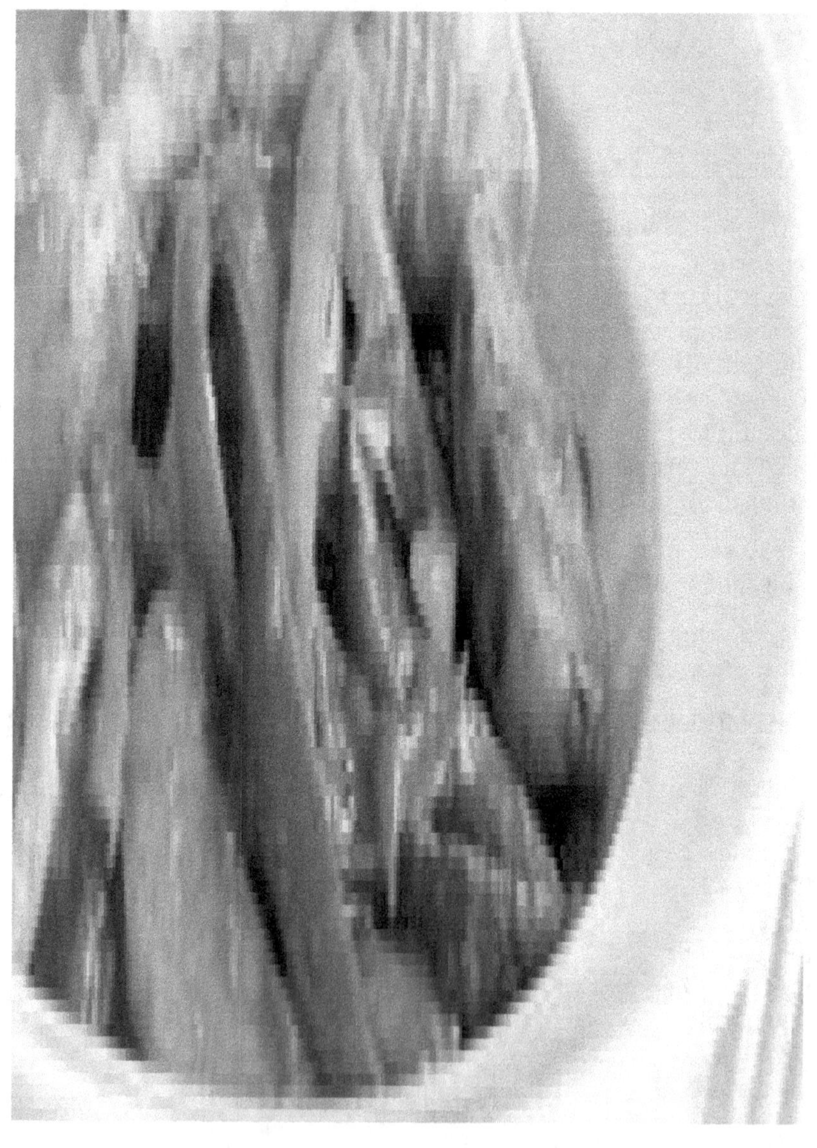

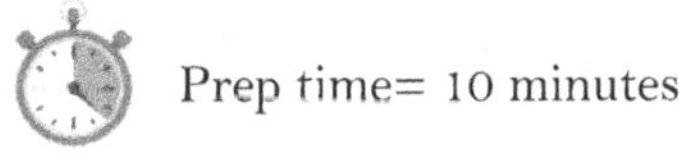 Prep time= 10 minutes

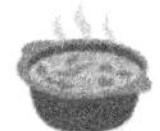 Cooking time= 25 minutes

INGREDIENTS

Olive oil, one tablespoon
3 cut and deseeded mixed peppers
400g of unpeeled baby potatoes and 1 large onion, thinly sliced
1 teaspoon smoked paprika
2 chopped garlic cloves
1 teaspoon dried thyme
400 g of canned diced tomatoes
4 fillets of salmon
1 tablespoon of parsley, chopped, to serve

Nutrient Unit

Kcal: 413
Fat: 18.9g
Saturates 3.9g
Carbs: 28.9g
Sugars: 11g
Fiber: 4.9g
Protein: 33g
low in salt: 0.33g

INSTRUCTION

STEP 1
Add the peppers, onion, and potatoes to a wide pan of hot oil. Cook for 5-8 minutes, stirring frequently, or until golden. The tomatoes, garlic, thyme, and paprika are then added. Stir and cover while bringing to a boil, then reduce heat and simmer for 12 minutes. If the sauce is too thick, add a little water.
STEP 2
Season the stew, then place the salmon on top with the skin facing up. Put the top back on and boil the salmon for an additional 8 minutes, or until it is cooked through. If desired, garnish with parsley before serving.

One-pan salmon with roast asparagus

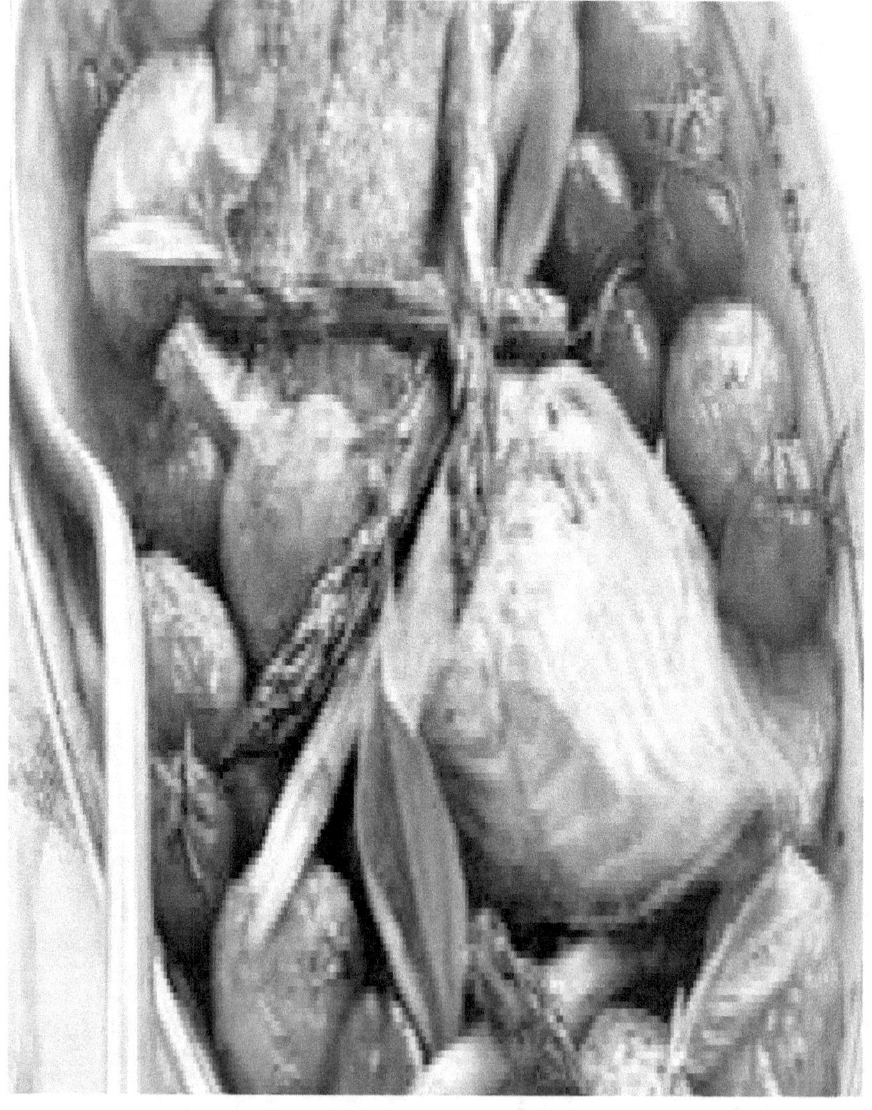

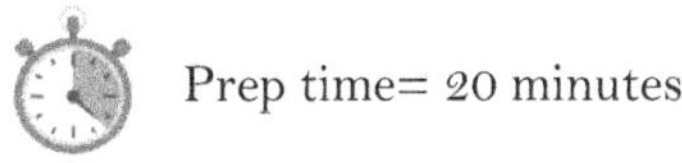 Prep time= 20 minutes

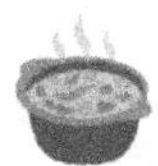 Cooking time= 50minutes

INGREDIENTS

400g new potato, halved if large
2 tbsp olive oil
8 asparagus spears, trimmed and halved
2 handfuls cherry tomatoes
1 tbsp balsamic vinegar
2 salmon fillets, about 140g/5oz each
handful basil leaves

Nutrient Unit

Kcal: 473
Fat: 24.5g
Saturates 3.8g
Carbs: 33.5g
Sugars: 5g
Fiber: 2.5g
Protein: 34g
low in salt: 0.25g

INSTRUCTION

STEP 1
Set oven to fan-forced 220°C and gas 7. Put 1 tablespoon of olive oil and the potatoes in an ovenproof dish, and roast for 20 minutes, or until the potatoes are beginning to brown. Place the potatoes and asparagus in the oven once again for 15 minutes
STEP 2
Add the cherry tomatoes, vinegar, and salmon, then mix everything. Return to the oven for an additional 10-15 minutes to finish cooking the salmon, then drizzle with the remaining oil. Serve everything straight from the plate after scattering the basil leaves over it.

Salmon and spinach with tartare cream

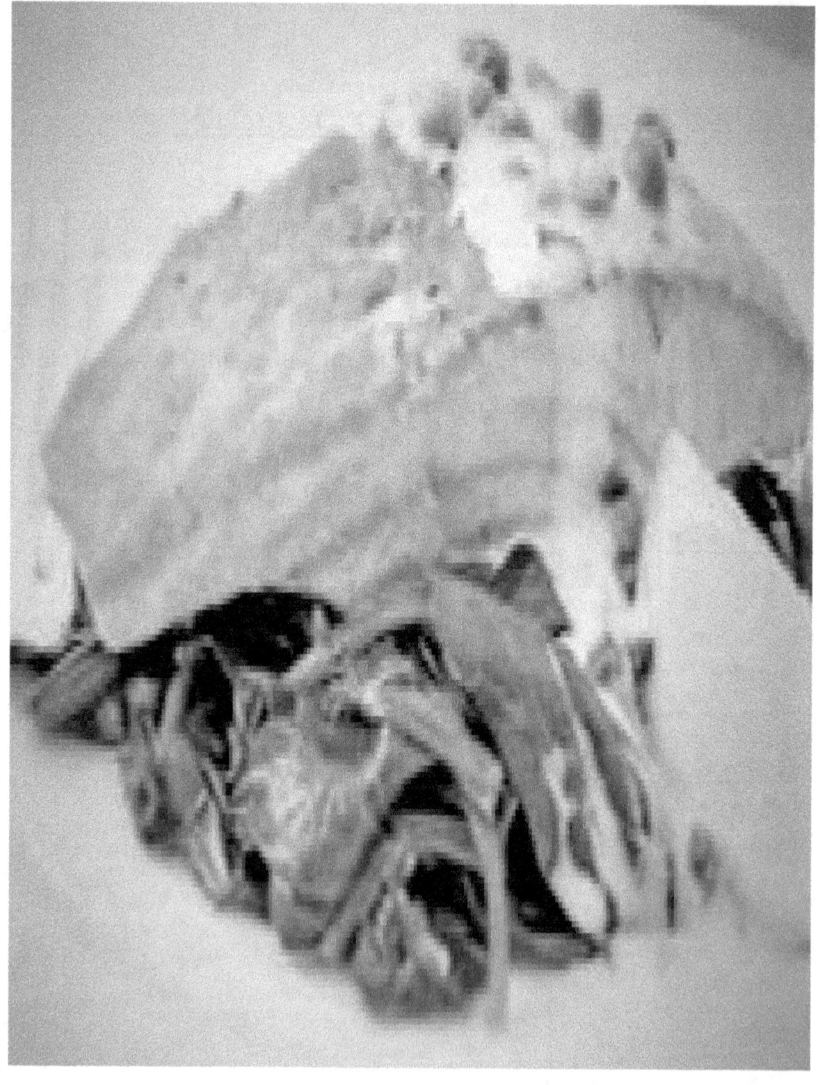

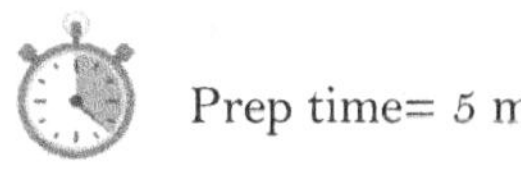 Prep time= 5 minutes

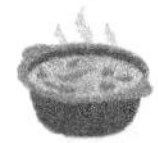 Cooking time= 10 minutes

INGREDIENTS

1 teaspoon of sunflower or vegetable oil
250g bag of spinach, 2 skinless salmon fillets
Reduced-fat crème fraiche
juice, 2 tablespoons ½ lemon
2 tablespoons flat-leaf parsley,
1 teaspoon drained capers, and lemon wedges for serving

Nutrient Unit

Kcal: 320
Fat: 19.6g
Saturates 6g
Carbs: 3.1g
Sugars: 3g
Fiber: 3.4g
Protein: 31g
low in salt: 0.67g

INSTRUCTION

STEP 1

Season the salmon on both sides with salt and pepper, then cook for 4 minutes on each side, or until brown and the flesh readily flakes. While the spinach is cooking, let the chicken rest on a platter.

STEP 2

Place the leaves in the hot pan, season them well, cover it, and let them wilt for one minute while stirring once or twice. Place the salmon on top of the spinach on the dishes. With a squeeze of lemon juice, capers, and parsley, warm the crème fraiche slowly in the pan. Then, add salt and pepper to taste. Don't let it boil, please. Serve the fish with the sauce on top and lemon wedges for dipping.

Lamb dopiaza with broccoli rice

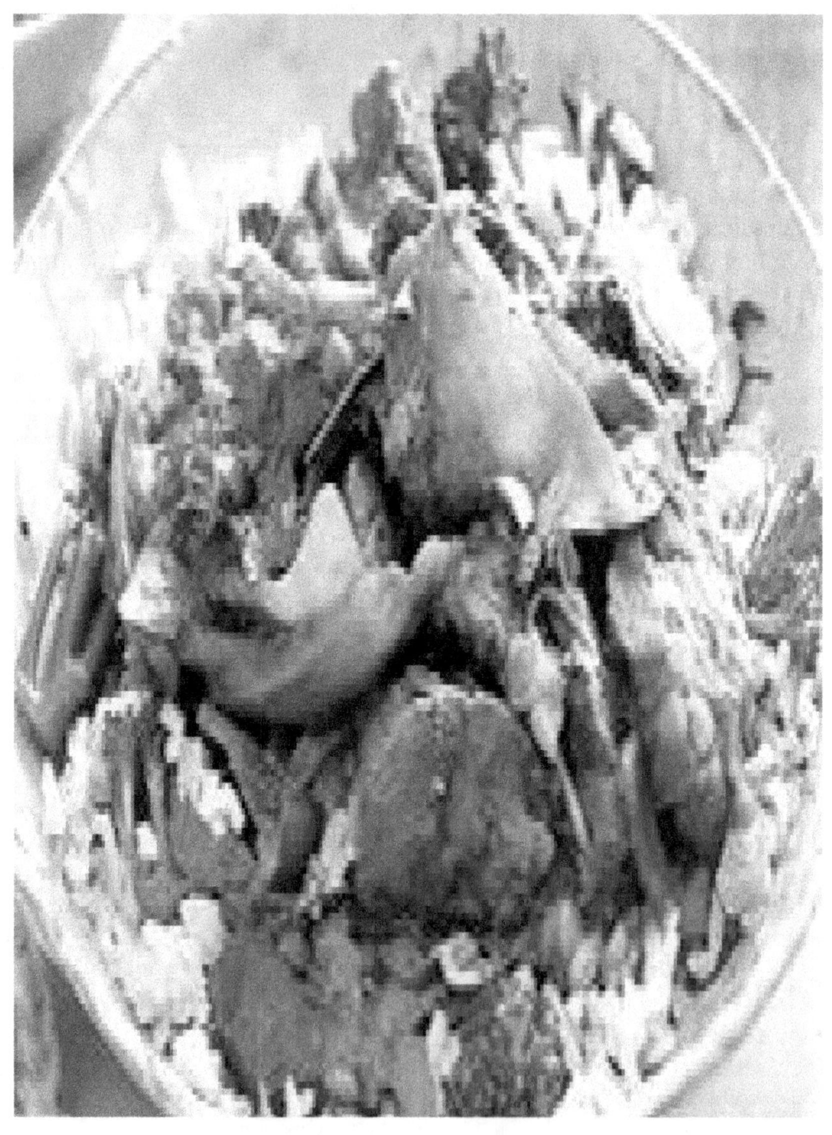

 Prep time= 20 minutes

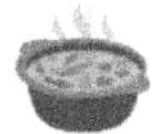 Cooking time= 1 hour 30 minutes

INGREDIENTS

lamb leg steaks weighing 225g, with the fat removed and chopped into 2.5 cm/ 1 in chunks.
50g full-fat organic bio yogurt plus 4 tablespoons to serve.
a tablespoon of medium curry powder
a teaspoon of cold-pressed rapeseed oil
2 medium onions, one thinly chopped and the other into five wedges.
2 peeled and thinly cut cloves of garlic
1 tablespoon peeled and chopped finely ginger
tiny broccoli florets weighing 100g
If you don't like it too spicy, de-seeded 1 little red chili
coarsely chopped 200g tomatoes
50g rinsed and dried split red lentils
coriander, coarsely chopped into a half-pack plus additional for garnish
a 100g package of baby spinach
Regarding the broccoli rice
100g brown whole-grain rice
tiny broccoli florets weighing

100g

Nutrient Unit

Kcal: 570
Fat: 13.7g
Saturates 3.6g
Carbs: 66g
Sugars: 13.5g
Fiber: 11.6g
Protein: 36g
low in salt: 0.32g

INSTRUCTION

STEP 1
Place the lamb in a big bowl and generously sprinkle with freshly ground black pepper. Stir well to incorporate before adding the yogurt and 1/2 tsp of the curry powder.

STEP 2
Warm up half the oil in a sizable nonstick pan. For 4-5 minutes, or until lightly browned and slightly tender, fry the onion wedges over high heat. Pour onto a platter, set aside, and then put the pan back on the stove.

STEP 3
Stirring regularly, add the remaining oil along with the sliced onions, garlic, ginger, and chili. Cover the pan and cook for 10 minutes, or until the ingredients are very soft. When the onions are beginning to turn brown, remove the lid, turn the heat up, and cook for an additional 2-3 minutes. This will give a ton of flavor, but watch out that they don't burn.

STEP 4
Once the heat has been reduced once more, add the tomatoes and remaining curry powder.

Cook for one minute, then add the yogurt and lamb to the pan and cook, stirring often, for four to five minutes at medium-high heat.

STEP 5
Pour 300 ml of cold water into the pan, add the lentils and coriander, stir, and cover with a lid. Cook on low heat for 45 minutes; the sauce should be boiling slowly. If the curry seems a bit dry, add a little more water. Stir the curry and remove the lid every 10-15 minutes.

STEP 6
After the curry has cooked for 30 minutes, cook the rice for 25 minutes, or until it is just soft, in plenty of boiling water. For an additional 3 minutes, add the broccoli florets. Do a good job of draining.

STEP 7
Take off the cover from the curry, add the reserved onion wedges, and simmer for a further 15 minutes or so, stirring frequently, or until the lamb is cooked. Add the spinach, a handful at a time, right before serving and allow it to wilt. Rice with broccoli and yogurt is served with coriander.

Turmeric smoothie bowl

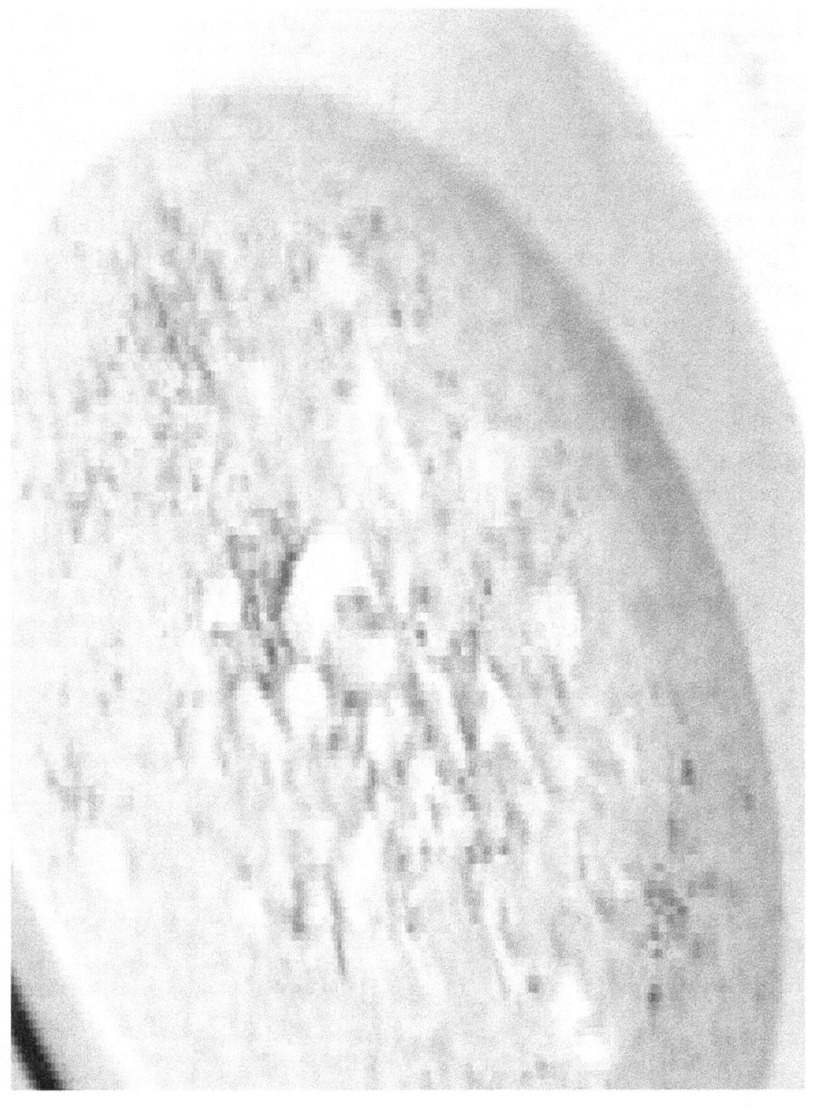

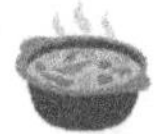 Prep time= 10 minutes

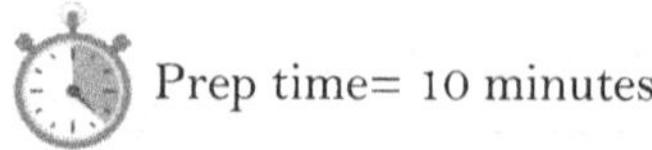 Cooking time= No

INGREDIENTS

10cm/4in of fresh turmeric or
2 tsp of crushed turmeric.
3 tablespoons coconut milk
yogurt (we used Co Yo), or the
cream removed from coconut
milk in a can.
50g of oats without gluten
1 tablespoon cashew butter or a
small amount of cashews
2 bananas, roughly sliced after
being peeled
1/2 tsp. of ground cinnamon
To serve, 1 tablespoon of
chopped nuts or chia seeds

Nutrient Unit

Kcal: 289
Fat: 9.5g
Saturates 3.9g
Carbs: 39.9g
Sugars: 19g
Fiber: 4.7g
Protein: 6g
low in salt: 0.01g

INSTRUCTION

STEP
If using, peel and grate the
turmeric root. Blend all
ingredients in a blender with
600ml of water until they are
completely smooth. Serve in a
bowl with some chopped nuts
or chia seeds on top.

Tikka-style fish

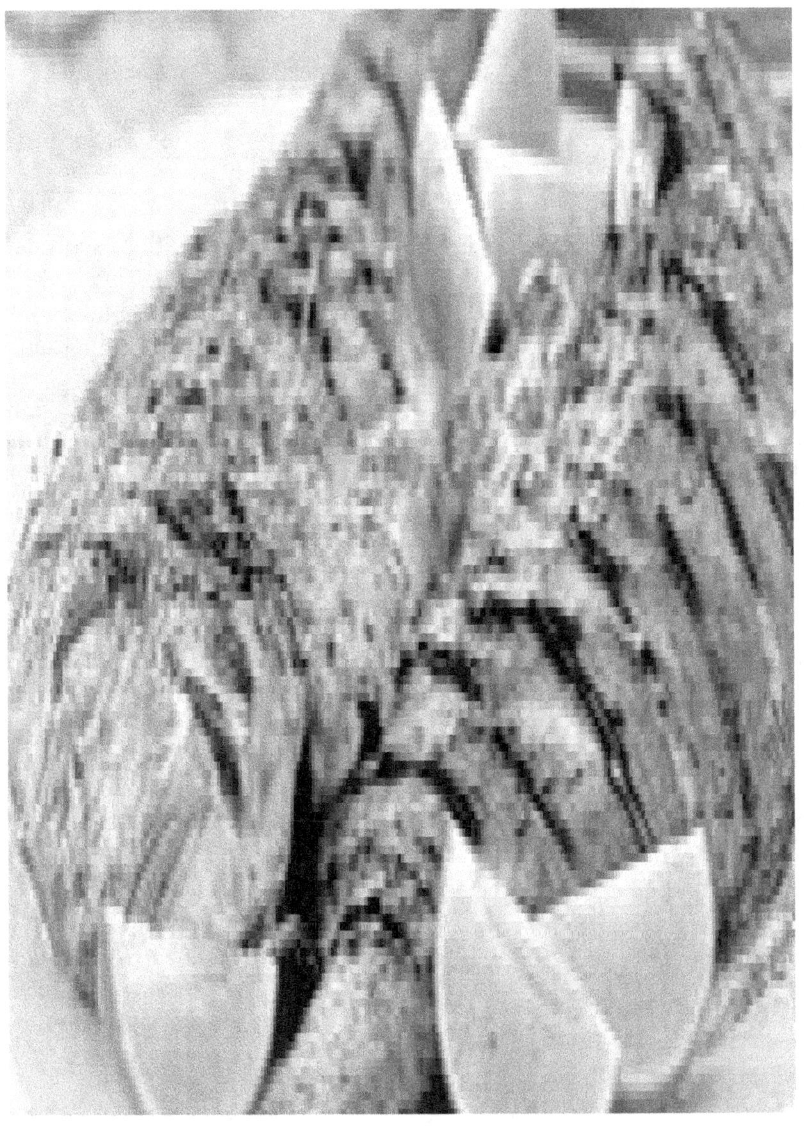

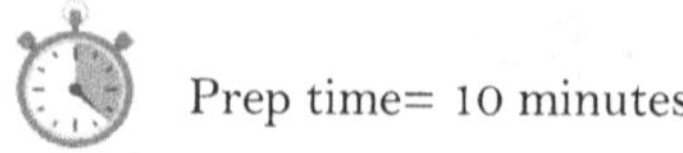 Prep time= 10 minutes

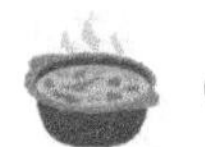 Cooking time= 15 minutes

INGREDIENTS

2 tablespoons of fresh root ginger, coarsely grated
4 garlic cloves, smashed or finely grated
2 red snapper or sea bream whole fish (each weighing about 900g/2lb) or 6 tuna steaks
Plain yogurt, six tablespoons
Olive oil, 2 tablespoons
Turmeric, 2 teaspoons
Mild chili powder, 2 teaspoons
Cumin seed, three tablespoons

Nutrient Unit

Kcal: 264
Fat: 10.9g
Saturates 1.9g
Carbs: 3.5g
Sugars: 1.1g
Fiber: 0g
Protein: 36g
low in salt: 0.65g

INSTRUCTION

STEP 1
Use a sharp knife to score the skin of the whole fish on both sides, if using. Rub the fish with a mixture of ginger and garlic, salt, and pepper.
STEP 2
Combine the yogurt, oil, seasoning, and spices. Use to coat the fish both internally and externally, then refrigerate until cooking time.
STEP 3
Cook the fish directly on the rack for 3–4 minutes for tuna steaks or 6–8 minutes for whole fish if you are concerned that it will adhere to the grill. How hot your barbecue is when you start cooking will determine how long it takes.

Spiced lamb kebabs with pea and herb couscous

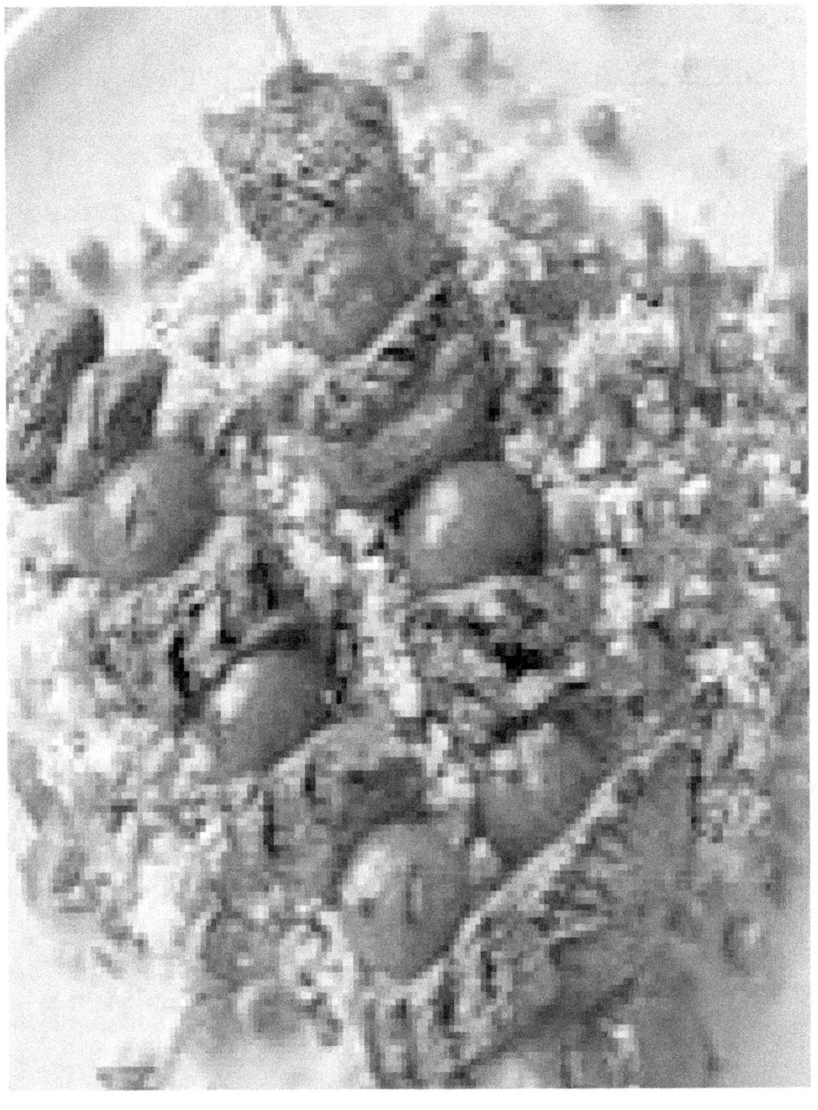

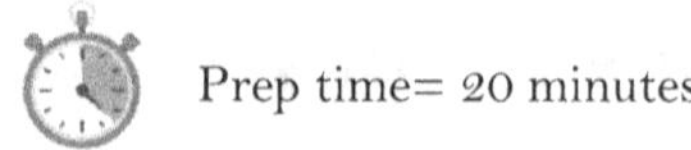 Prep time= 20 minutes

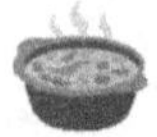 Cooking time= 20 minutes

INGREDIENTS	Nutrient Unit

INGREDIENTS

400g cubes of lean lamb
shoulder, sliced into thirds
1 teaspoon cumin powder
12 teaspoons cayenne pepper
One tablespoon of sweet
smoked paprika
Olive oil, 1 tablespoon
There are twenty-four cherry
tomatoes.
Couscous weight: 140 grams
400 ml of heated vegetable
broth
140 g frozen pea
juice, one large carrot, coarsely
shredded, a small pack of
coriander, chopped, a small
pack of mint, chopped. 1
lemon
2-tablespoons of extra virgin
olive oil

Nutrient Unit

Kcal: 455
Fat: 24g
Saturates 7.5g
Carbs: 34g
Sugars: 8g
Fiber: 6.5g
Protein: 27g
low in salt: 0.76g

<u>**INSTRUCTION**</u>

STEP 1
Soak 6 wooden skewers in water for 30 minutes to stop them from burning when used for grilling or griddling. Place the lamb cubes, spices, and olive oil in a large basin. Season and thoroughly combine everything.

STEP 2
Skewer a cherry tomato after placing a slice of lamb on it. Repeat the process, placing about 4 pieces of lamb and 4 cherry tomatoes on each skewer, and continue doing so until all are utilized.

STEP 3
In the meantime, put the couscous in a big bowl, add the boiling vegetable stock, and then stir in the peas. Stir and let soak for about five minutes before covering with cling film.

STEP 4
Preheat a griddle. When the couscous has absorbed all of the liquid, lightly fluff the grains with a fork before adding the carrot, herbs, lemon juice, and olive oil. Mix everything thoroughly, add the seasoning and reserve.

STEP 5
Cook the skewers on the hot griddle for 5 to 6 minutes, then flip them over and cook for an additional 5 to 6 minutes, or until the meat and tomatoes are scorched and well cooked. Along with the couscous, serve the skewers.

Chickpea stew with tomatoes and spinach

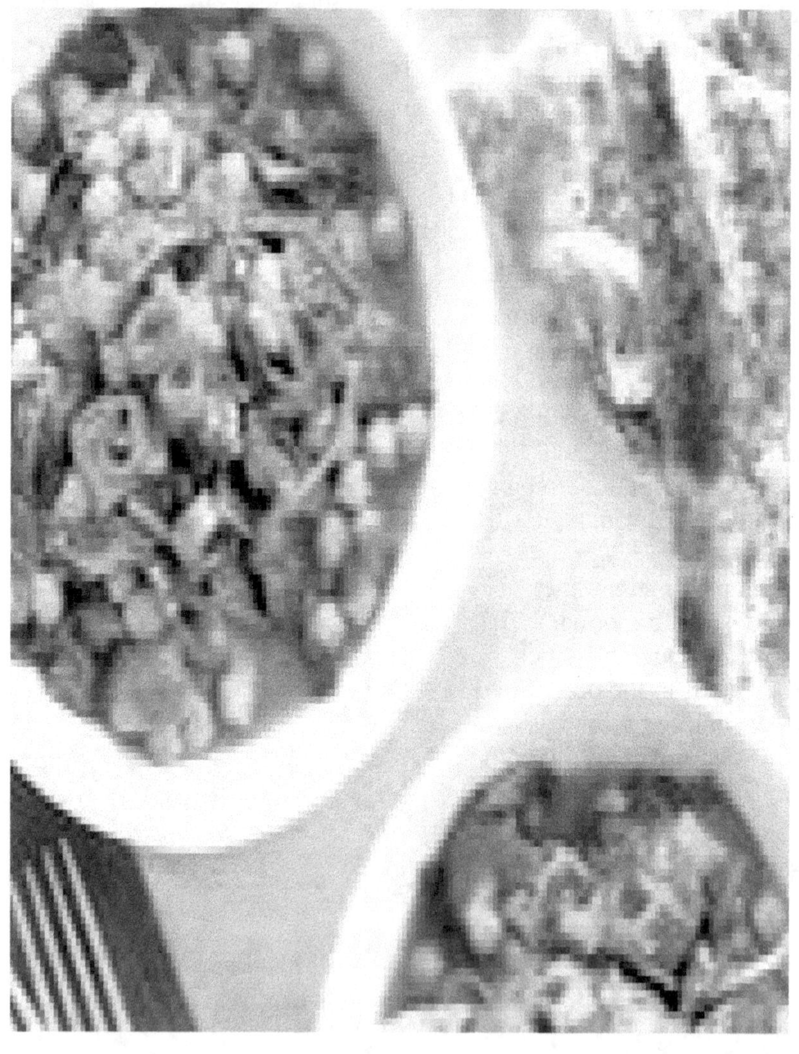

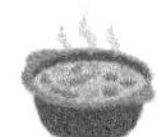 Prep time= 10 minutes

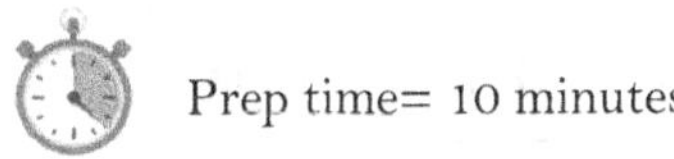 Cooking time= 25 minutes

INGREDIENTS

1-tablespoon vegetable oil
Sliced red onion, one
a finger-length piece of fresh
root ginger, shredded, and two
garlic cloves, diced.
1/2 teaspoon of turmeric and 2
mild red chilies, thinly sliced
3/4 teaspoon garam masala
1 teaspoon cumin, ground
four tomatoes cut up
1 teaspoon tomato puree
400 g can chickpea washed and
drained
200 g of young spinach leaves,
to be served with rice or naan
bread

Nutrient Unit

Kcal: 144
Fat: 5.6g
Saturates 0.01g
Carbs: 16.5g
Sugars: 5,7g
Fiber: 4.9g
Protein: 6.6g
low in salt: 0.57g

INSTRUCTION

STEP 1
Warm up the oil in a wok,
then sauté the onion until it
softens. Stirring often,
simmer for a further 5
minutes, or until the onions
are brown and the garlic is
just beginning to toast.
STEP 2
Stirring briefly over low heat,
add the cumin, garam masala,
and turmeric. Add the tomato
purée and chopped tomatoes,
then boil for five minutes.
STEP 3
Fill the chickpeas' can with
300 ml of water, then add
them to the pan. Before
stirring in the spinach to wilt,
simmer for 10 minutes. Serve
with rice after seasoning.

Pear and blueberry breakfast bowl

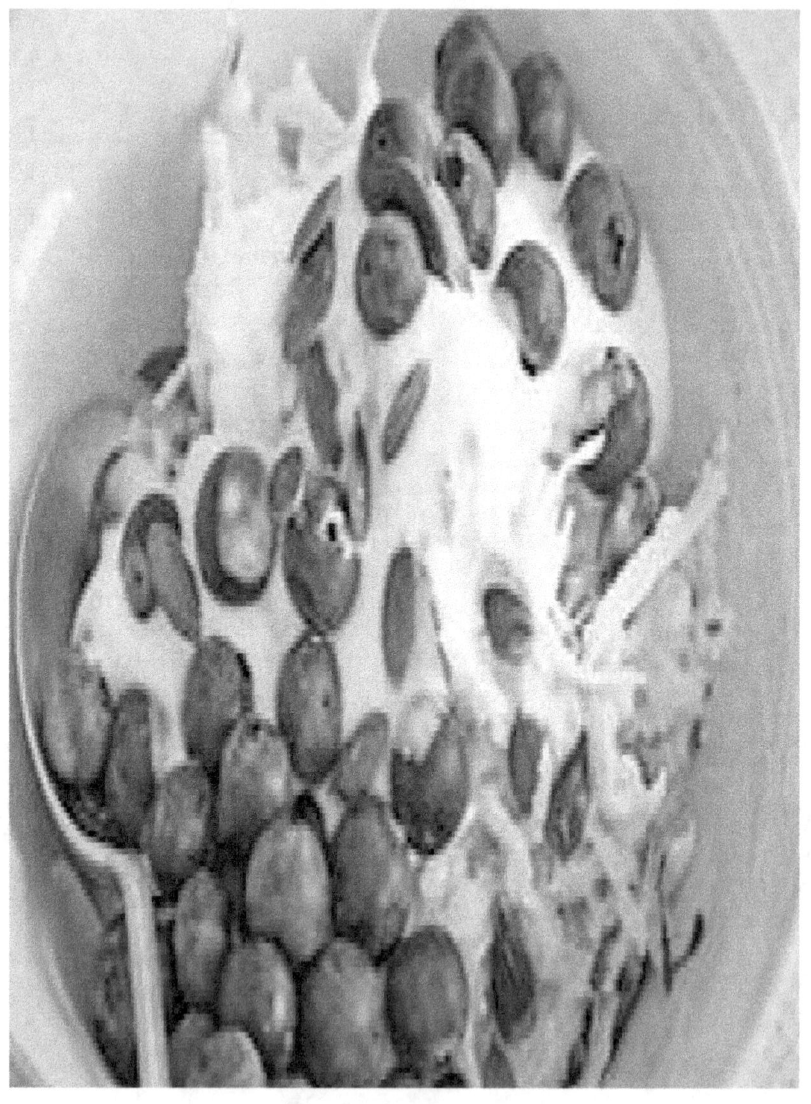

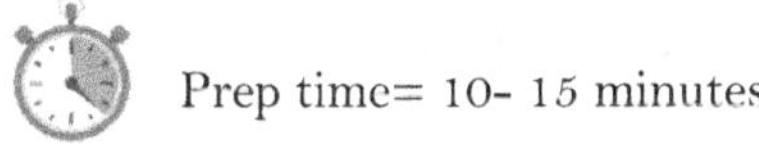 Prep time= 10- 15 minutes

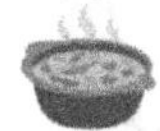 Cooking time= No

INGREDIENTS

1 pear with red skin that is firm
but ripe, unpeeled
two tablespoons of oats
150g pot 0% fat bioyogurt
a little bit more than 3
tablespoons of skim milk
1 tbsp. pumpkin seeds
2 sacks of blueberries

Nutrient Unit

Kcal: 414
Fat: 8.9g
Saturates 1.9g
Carbs: 56g
Sugars: 37g
Fiber: 10.9g
Protein: 19.5g
low in salt: 0.26g

INSTRUCTION

STEP 1
Grate the pear and mix it with
the oats, milk, milk and half of
the yogurt in a bowl. After
waiting for 5 to 10 minutes,
check the consistency and, if
necessary, thin with a little
more milk or water. The
remaining yogurt should be
spooned on, followed by a
heap of the berries and seeds.

Homemade granola

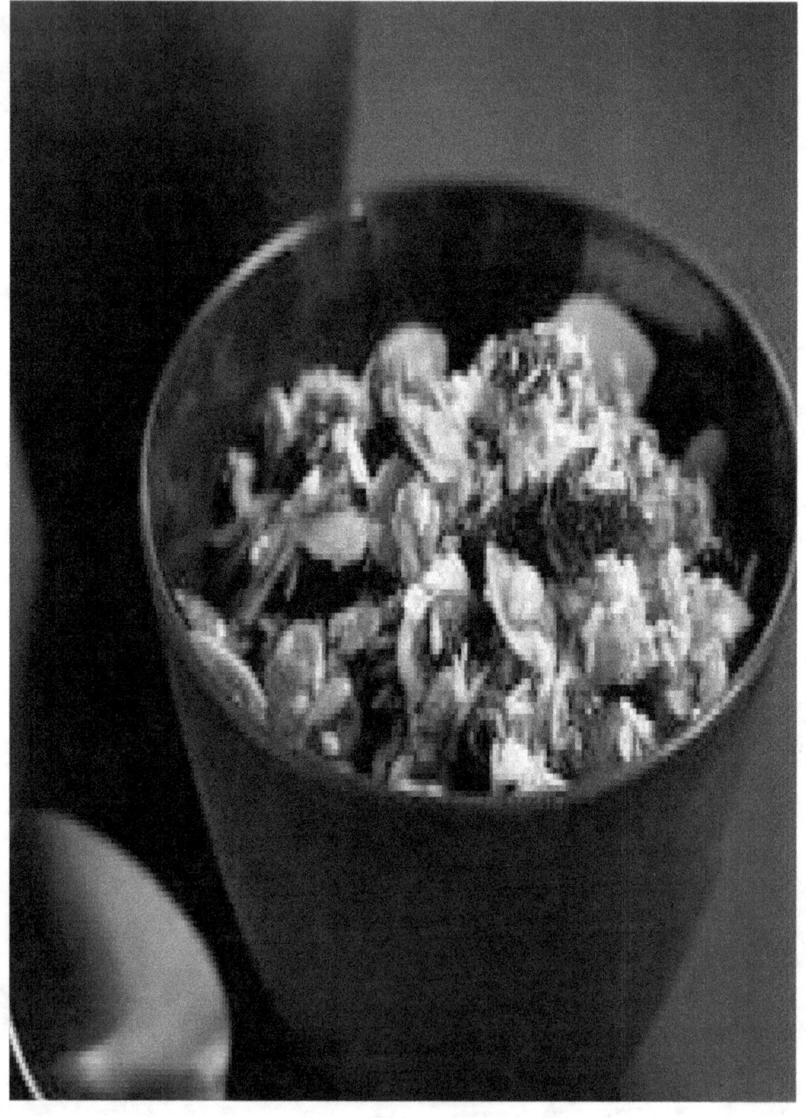

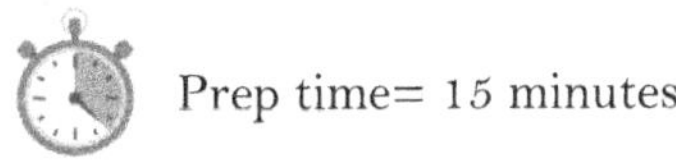 Prep time= 15 minutes

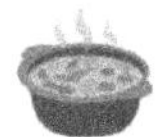 Cooking time= 25 minutes

INGREDIENTS

Vegetable oil, two tablespoons
Maple syrup, 125 milliliters
Honey, two tablespoons
1 tablespoon vanilla extract
Rolling Oats, 300g
100 sunflower seeds
4 tbsp. sesame seeds
50 g of pumpkin seeds
100g of flaked almond
100g dried berries, available in
the baking section
50g desiccated coconut or
coconut flakes

Nutrient Unit

Kcal: 257
Fat: 14.9g
Saturates 3.1g
Carbs: 27.9g
Sugars: 12.8g
Fiber: 2.6g
Protein: 5g
low in salt: 0.02g

INSTRUCTION

STEP 1

Oven temperature: 150°C/fan 130°C/gas 2. In a big bowl, combine the oil, maple syrup, honey, and vanilla. Except for the dried fruit and coconut, add the remaining ingredients and thoroughly combine.

STEP 2

Spread the granola equally after being tipped onto two baking sheets. After 15 minutes of baking, add the coconut and dried fruit, and bake for an additional 10 to 15 minutes. To cool, remove and scrape onto a flat tray. Serve with yogurt or cold milk. For up to a month, the granola can be kept in an airtight container.

Bean and barley soup

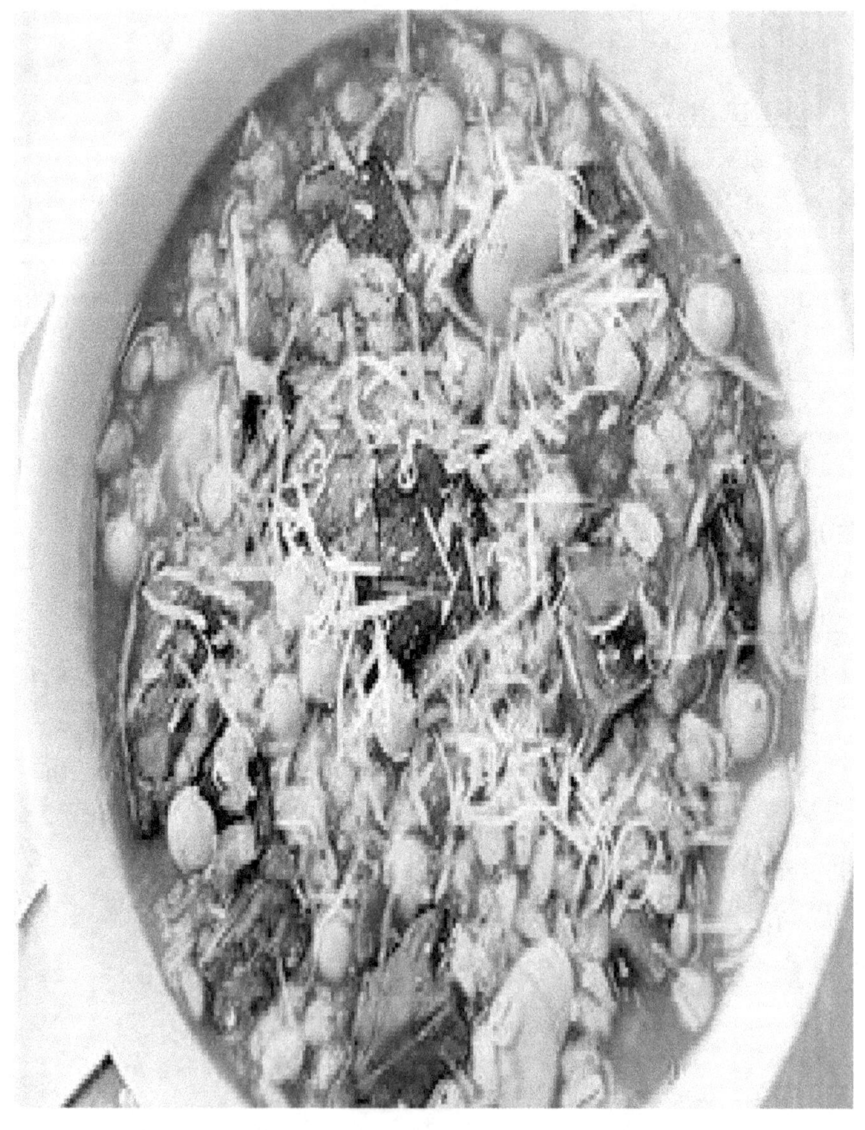

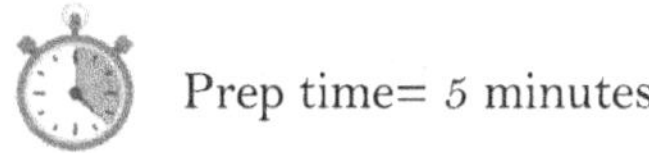 Prep time= 5 minutes

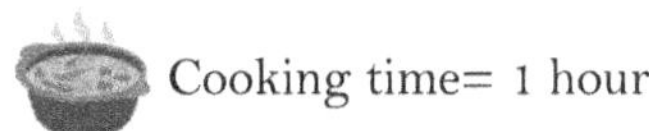 Cooking time= 1 hour

INGREDIENTS

2 tablespoons of vegetable oil
1 big onion, diced finely
1 cut, quartered, and cored
fennel bulb
5 smashed garlic cloves
400 g can of washed and drained
chickpeas
400g cans of chopped tomatoes
in two
a liter of vegetable stock
250g of pearl rye
215g can of rinsed and drained
butter beans
100g of grated parmesan-topped
baby spinach leaves.

Nutrient Unit

Kcal: 376
Fat: 13.9g
Saturates 1.2g
Carbs: 48.9g
Sugars: 4.5g
Fiber: 6.9g
Protein: 11g
low in salt: 0.13g

INSTRUCTION

STEP 1

Onion, fennel, and garlic should
be cooked in oil for 10 to 12
minutes, or until they are tender
and starting to brown, in a
medium saucepan over medium
heat.

STEP 2

When adding the tomatoes,
stock, and barley to the pan,
mash half of the chickpeas. Add
more water to the top and bring
to a boil. Then, turn the heat
down and simmer, covered, for
45 minutes, or until the barley is
soft. If the liquid is much
decreased, add another can of
water

STEP 3

The soup should be
supplemented with the
remaining chickpeas and butter
beans. Add the spinach and cook
for about a minute, or until it
wilts, a few minutes have
passed. Sprinkle Parmesan on
top after seasoning.

Barley, broccoli risotto with lemon and basil

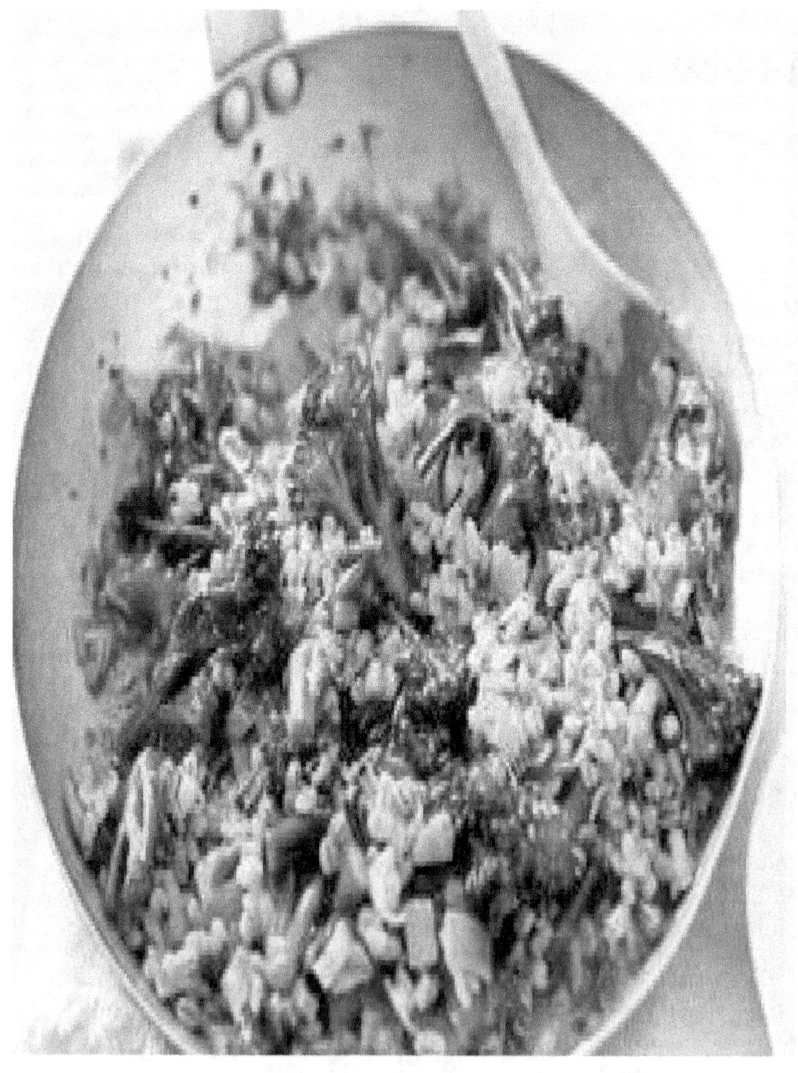

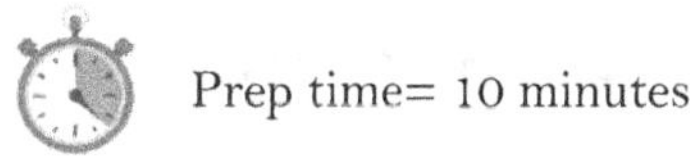 Prep time= 10 minutes

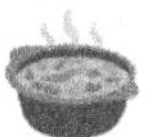 Cooking time= 35 minutes

INGREDIENTS

100 grams of whole-grain
pearl barley
2 tablespoons powdered
vegetable bouillon with
reduced salt
two tablespoons of rapeseed
oil
Chopped one sizable leek
two garlic cloves.
2/3 a pack of basil, generously
squeezed lemon juice
from a 200g pack, 125g of
tender stem broccoli

Nutrient Unit

Kcal: 486
Fat: 8.9g
Saturates 1g
Carbs: 77.9g
Sugars: 10.9g
Fiber: 12g
Protein: 15g
low in salt: 1.36g

INSTRUCTION

STEP 1
Overnight soaking of the barley is
accomplished by covering it with
one liter of cold water.
STEP 2
Drain the barley the following day
and save the liquid to make 500ml
of vegetable bouillon. The leek
should be cooked for a little while
to soften in a nonstick pan with
the remaining oil heated. Pour
half of the mixture into a bowl,
then stir in the barley and
bouillon. Put the lid on and
simmer for 20 minutes.
STEP 3
Meanwhile, add the garlic, basil,
remaining oil, lemon juice, and 3
tbsp water to the leeks in the dish,
and blitz to a paste with a stick
blender
STEP 4
The broccoli should be added to
the pan after the barley has
cooked for 20 minutes and should
be simmered for an additional 5 to
10 minutes to make both soft.
Add the puréed basil and cook it
just long enough to keep the aroma.

Tangy roast pepper and walnut dip

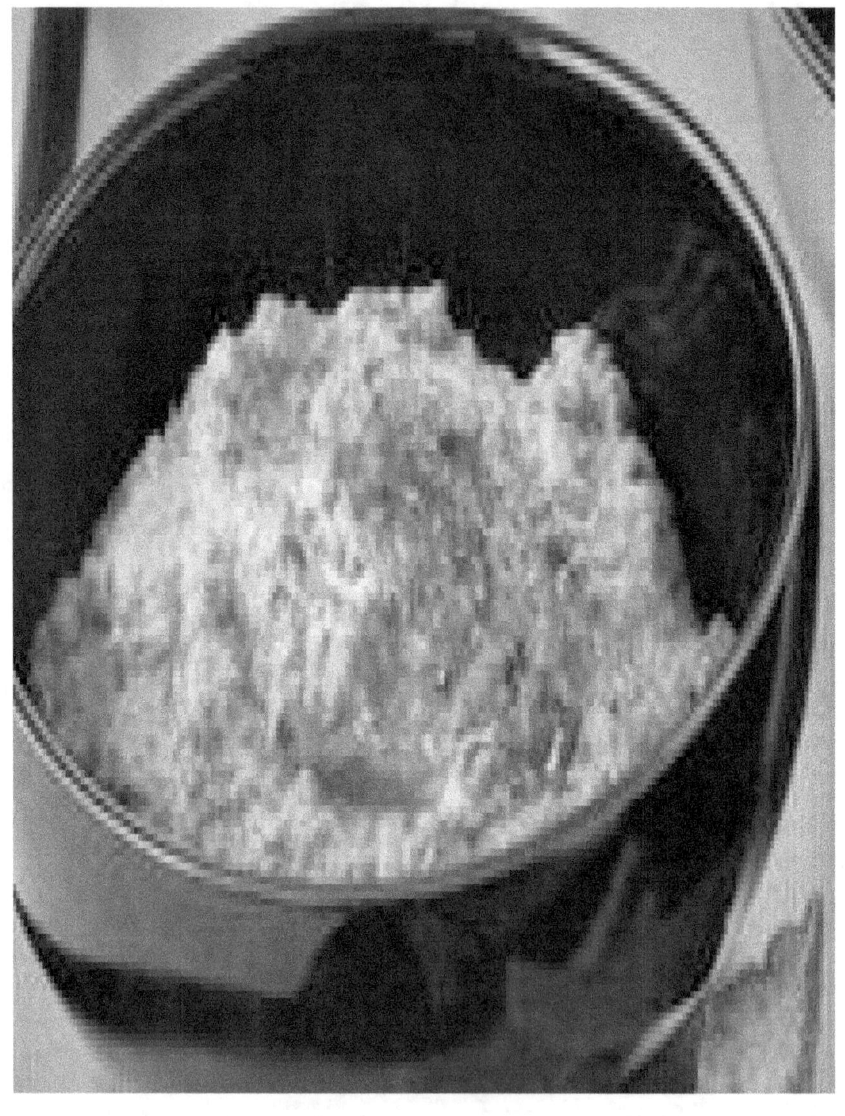

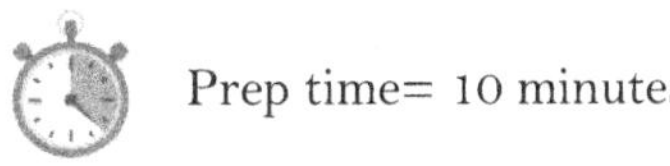 Prep time= 10 minutes

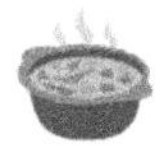 Cooking time= 2 minutes

INGREDIENTS

1 teaspoon of ground cumin and
1 teaspoon of ground pimento
(smoked paprika), plus
additional for serving
6 tablespoons of extra virgin
olive oil
100g walnut half-shells
225 grams of roasted red pepper,
drained, from a jar
1 tablespoon tomato purée
single smashed garlic clove
Lemon juice or red wine vinegar
may be used in place of the two
tablespoons of pomegranate
molasses.

Nutrient Unit

Kcal: 196
Fat: 17g
Saturates 1.9g
Carbs: 6.9g
Sugars: 4.51g
Fiber: 0.01g
Protein: 1.9g
low in salt: 0.38g

INSTRUCTION

STEP 1
The pimento and cumin
powder should be heated in
olive oil until aromatic in a
skillet. Salt and pepper to
taste, then combine the
remaining ingredients in a
food processor. Slowly add the
spiced oil while the motor is
running until it is combined.
Should it be too thick, add a
tablespoon of water. Pimento
and freshly ground black
pepper should be sprinkled on
top after scooping into a dish.

Winter leaf and parsnip salad with walnuts

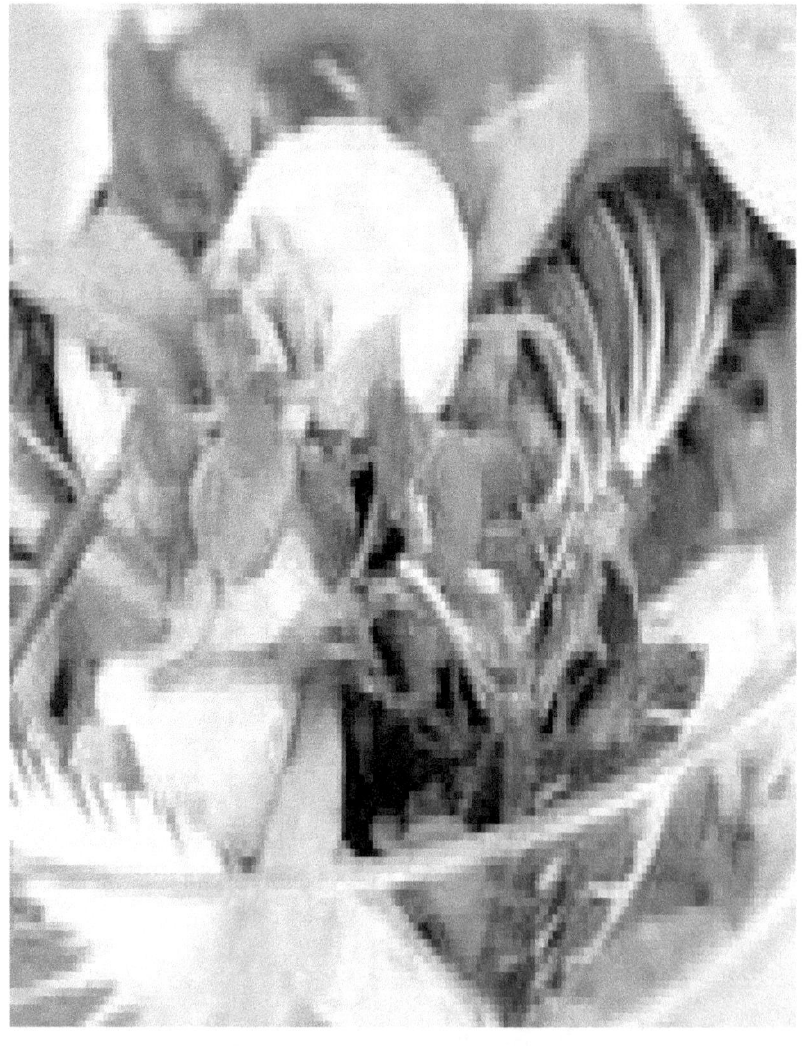

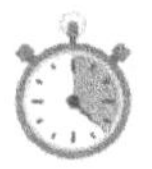 Prep time= 10 minutes

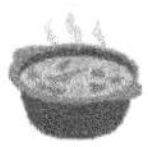 Cooking time= 25 minutes

INGREDIENTS

1 cm rounds of 4 parsnips, sliced
two tablespoons of vegetable oil
100g walnut half-shells
Separated leaves on three huge heads of chicory or radicchio
200 grams of a mixture of salad leaves, such as watercress and baby spinach

Nutrient Unit

Kcal: 134
Fat: 10.9g
Saturates 1g
Carbs: 7.9g
Sugars: 4g
Fiber: 2.9g
Protein: 3.1g
low in salt: 0.03g

INSTRUCTION

STEP 1

preheat the oven to 200°C/180°F fan/gas 6. Roast the parsnips for 20 to 25 minutes, or until golden and tender, after tossing them in the oil in a roasting pan. The nuts should be colored after an additional 15 minutes of roasting after adding them. Exit the oven, then let cool. up to two days before cooking.

STEP 2

A sizable serving bowl should contain all the leaves, parsnips, and nuts.

STEP 3

The vinaigrette should be prepared using the instructions below and served on the side so that guests may add their own dressing and the salad will not go soggy if it is not consumed right away.

Mustardy beetroot and lentil salad

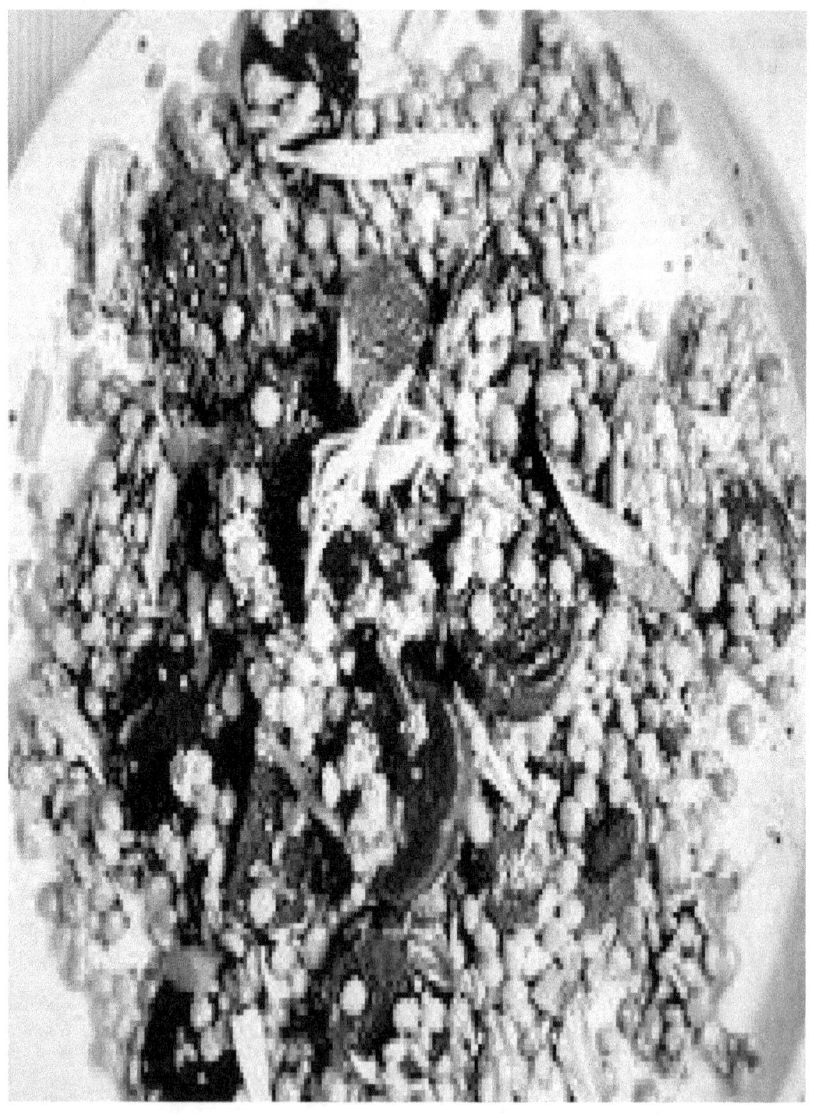

 Prep time= 5 minutes

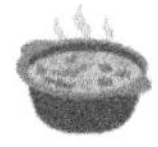 Cooking time= 20 minutes

INGREDIENTS

200 grams of puy lentils (or use two 250-gram packages of pre-cooked lentils)
1 tablespoon whole-grain mustard (or a substitute made without gluten)
1 1/2 tbsp extra virgin olive oil
A sliced huge handful of tarragon coarsely chopped
300g pack of cooked beetroot (not in vinegar).

Nutrient Unit

Kcal: 155
Fat: 3.9g
Saturates 1g
Carbs: 20.9g
Sugars: 5.7g
Fiber: 6g
Protein: 9.9g
low in salt: 0.31g

INSTRUCTION

STEP 1

Lentils should be cooked as directed on the package if you aren't using pre-cooked lentils, then drained and allowed to cool. While waiting, prepare a dressing by combining mustard, oil, and some seasoning.

STEP 2

Pour the dressing over the lentils in a bowl, then combine thoroughly. Serve after adding some spice, the tarragon, and the beetroot.

Tortellini with pesto and broccoli

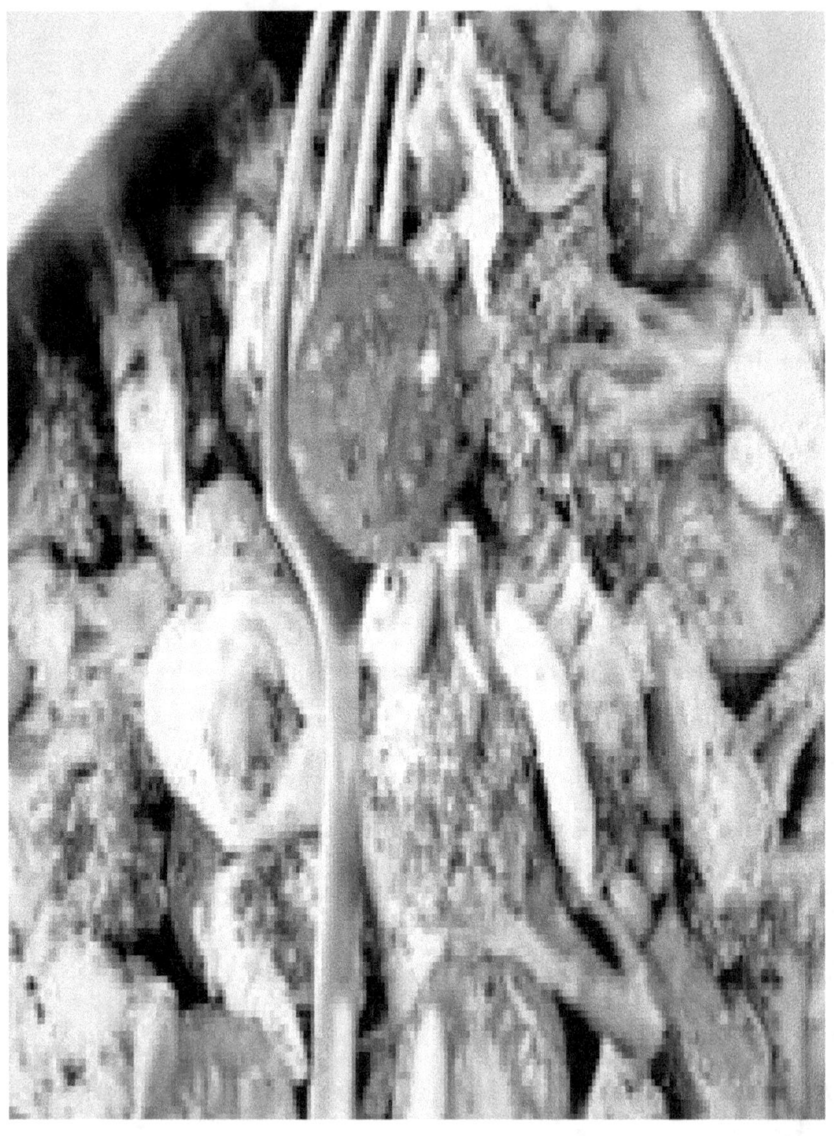

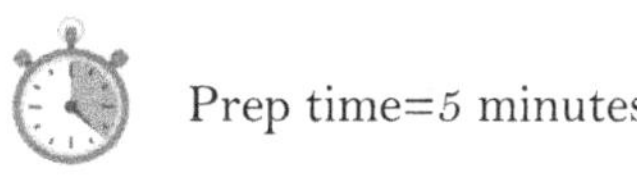 Prep time=5 minutes

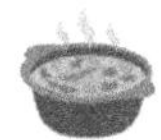 Cooking time=5 minutes

INGREDIENTS

140 grams of short-cut tender-stem broccoli
250 grams of new tortellini
if you can, use fresh pesto, 3 tbsp.
2 tablespoons roasted pine nuts
balsamic vinegar, 1 tablespoon
Halved cherry tomatoes, eight

Nutrient Unit

Kcal: 571
Fat: 25.9g
Saturates 8.9g
Carbs: 28.9g
Sugars: 11g
Fiber: 4.9g
Protein: 33g
low in salt: 0.33g

INSTRUCTION

STEP 1

Activate the stovetop to boil water in a big pan. Tortellini should be prepared as directed on the package, usually 2 minutes after the broccoli and 2 minutes after the tortellini. Drain everything, give it a gentle rinse in cold water until it cools, and then pour it all into a basin. Pine nuts, pesto, and balsamic vinegar should be added before tossing. Place the tomatoes in the mix, then chill the containers. For the tomatoes and pesto to impart their most flavor, let the salad come to room temperature in the morning.

Spanish spinach omelet

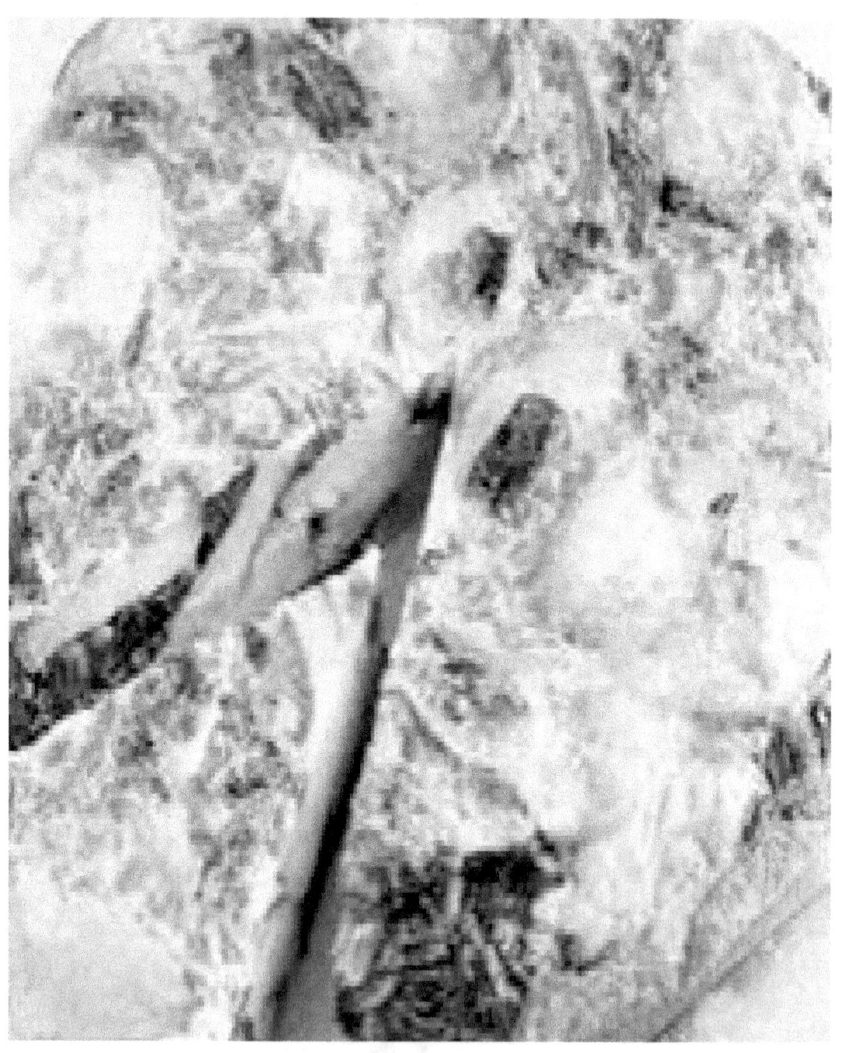

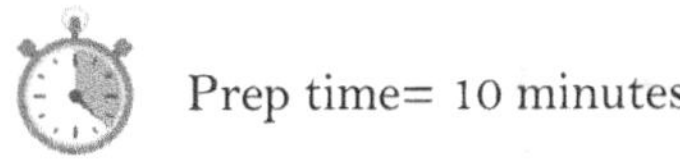 Prep time= 10 minutes

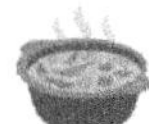 Cooking time=30 minutes

INSTRUCTION

INGREDIENTS

spinach greens in a 400g bag
Olive oil, 3 tablespoons
one big onion, thinly sliced
Peeled and thinly sliced two
big potatoes
10 eggs

Nutrient Unit

Kcal: 207
Fat: 12.9g
Saturates 3. g
Carbs: 10.9g
Sugars: 2g
Fiber: 1.9g
Protein: 12g
low in salt: 0.43g

STEP 1

Put a saucepan of water on to boil as you empty the spinach into a big colander. To wilt the spinach, slowly pour the water over it. Next, chill the spinach with cold water. Put the spinach in a strainer and squeeze out all the moisture.

STEP 2

the grill is really hot. For about 10 minutes, or until the potato is soft, gently sauté the onion and potato in oil in a nonstick frying pan. The eggs should be beaten together in a big basin with salt and pepper while the onion is frying. Stir the spinach into the potatoes before adding the eggs. Cook the omelette, stirring periodically, until nearly set, then quickly broil the top to set it. Flip the omelette over and place it back in the pan after easing it onto a platter. Turn the omelette out onto a board after the underside has finished cooking. Serve the food in wedges.

Vegan banana bread

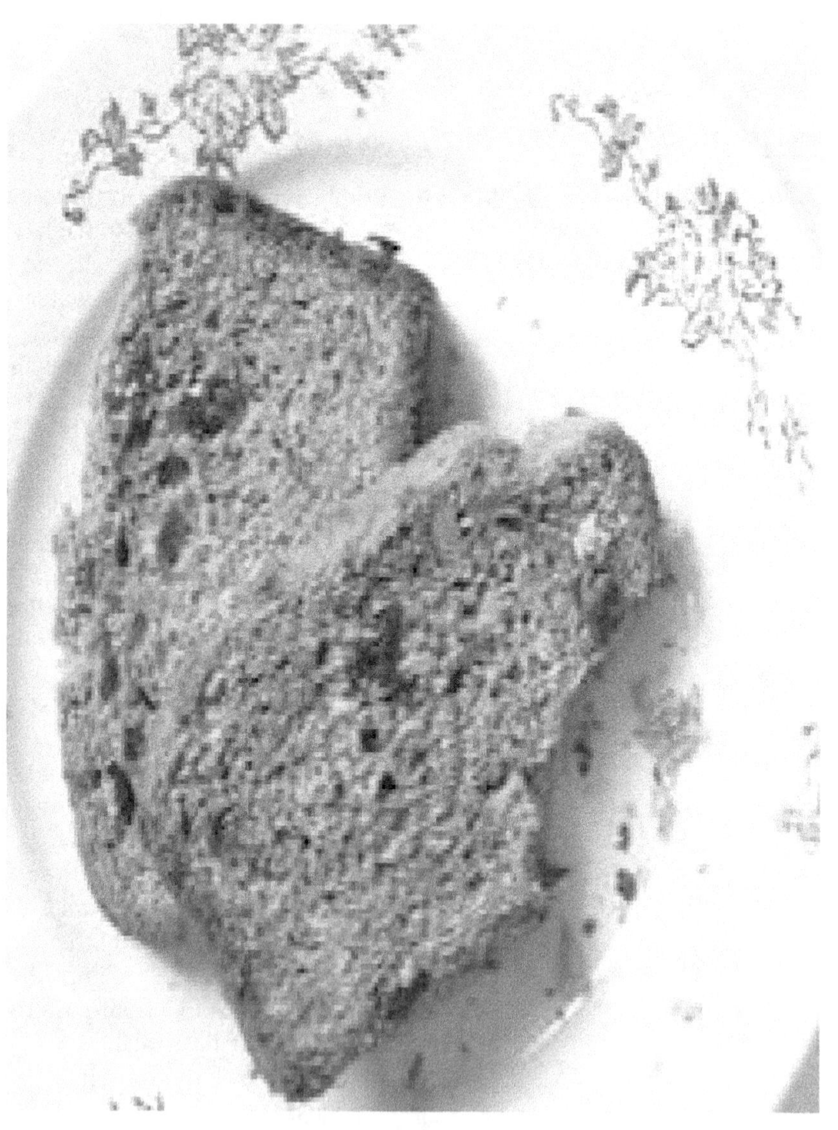

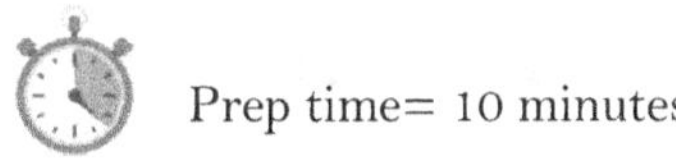 Prep time= 10 minutes

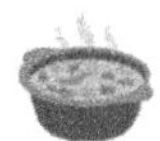 Cooking time= 40 minutes

INGREDIENTS

3 substantial bananas, black
75 ml of vegetable or
sunflower oil plus additional
for the tin
1 kg brown sugar
225 grams of normal flour (or
substitute self-rising flour and
cut the baking powder in half
to 2 heaping teaspoons)
3-tablespoon-full of baking
powder
3 teaspoons cinnamon or
mixed spices
fifty grams of optional dried
fruit or nuts

Nutrient Unit

Kcal: 217
Fat: 8g
Saturates 1g
Carbs: 32.9g
Sugars: 14g
Fiber: 2.9g
Protein: 3g
low in salt: 0.45g

INSTRUCTION

STEP 1

the oven to 200°C/180°F/gas 6.
3 large black bananas that have
been peeled and mashed with a
fork are combined with 100g of
brown sugar and 75g of
vegetable or sunflower oil.

STEP 2

Add 3 heaping tsp baking
powder, 3 tsp cinnamon or
mixed spices, and 225g of
ordinary flour and stir well.
Including 50g of nuts or dried
fruit is optional.

STEP 3

20 minutes of baking in a 2 lb
loaf pan that has been lined with
oil. If the cake is browning,
check and cover it with foil.

STEP 4

If a spear comes out clean, bake
for an additional 20 minutes.
Before cutting, give it some time
to cool. Despite having a nice
gooey quality, the next day, it is
still great when it is first baked.

Sweet potato and peanut curry

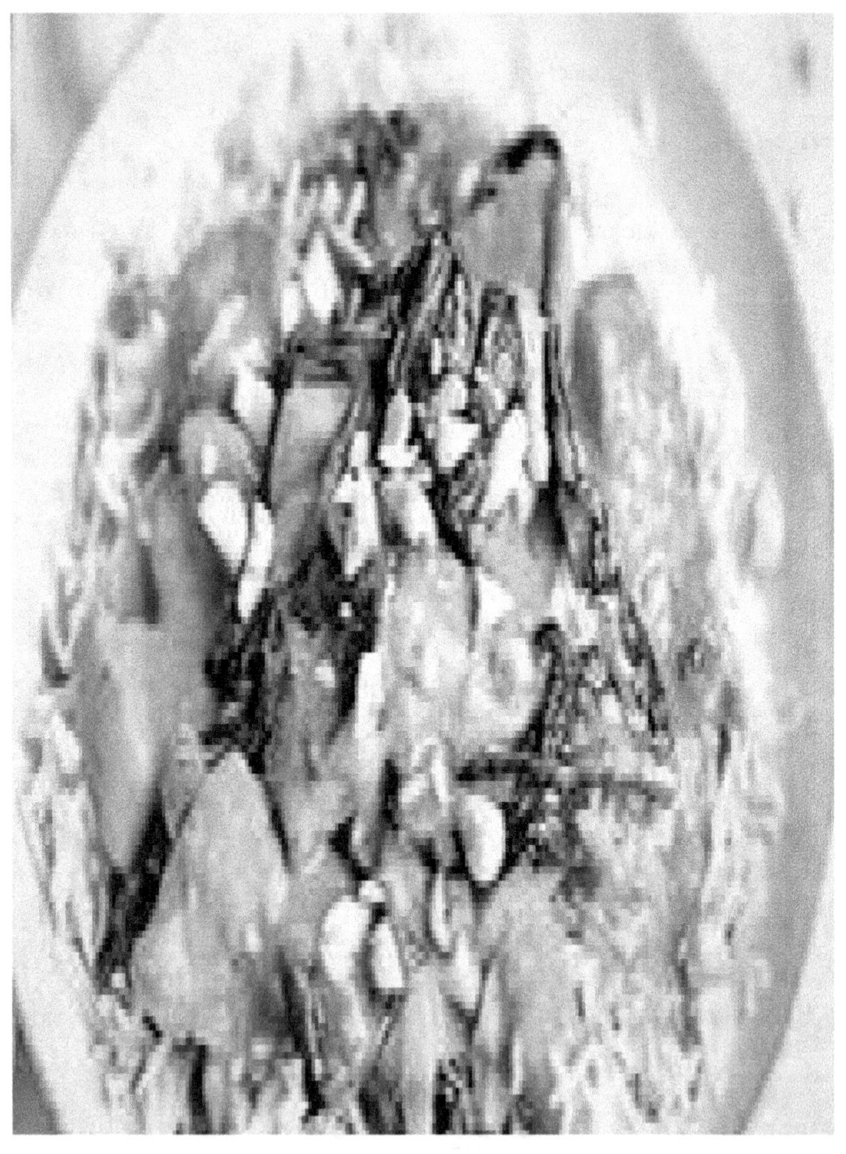

 Prep time= 15 minutes

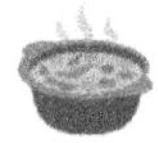 Cooking time= 45 minutes

INGREDIENTS

1-tablespoon coconut oil
1 chopped onion, 2 grated
garlic cloves, 1 small piece of
grated ginger
3 tablespoons Thai red curry
paste (check the label to see if
it's vegan or vegetarian)
1 tablespoon creamy peanut
butter
500 grams of sweet potatoes,
chunked after being skinned
Can of coconut milk, 400 ml.

Nutrient Unit

Kcal: 385
Fat: 24g
Saturates 17.9g
Carbs: 31.9g
Sugars: 14g
Fiber: 6.9g
Protein: 5g
low in salt: 0.5g

INSTRUCTION

STEP 1
One chopped onion should be
softened for five minutes in one
tablespoon of melted coconut oil
over medium heat. One minute
later, add two grated garlic
cloves and a piece of grated
ginger about the size of your
thumb.
STEP 2
Add 400 ml coconut milk and
200 ml water after stirring in 3
tbsp Thai red curry paste, 1 tbsp
smooth peanut butter, and 500 g
of peeled and chopped sweet
potatoes.
STEP 3
Bring to a boil, lower the heat,
cover the pot, and simmer for
25–30 minutes, or until the
sweet potato is tender.
STEP 4
Season well after adding 200g of
spinach and 1 lime juice. Serve
with cooked rice and top with a
few dry-roasted peanuts if you'd
like some crunch.

Berry omelet

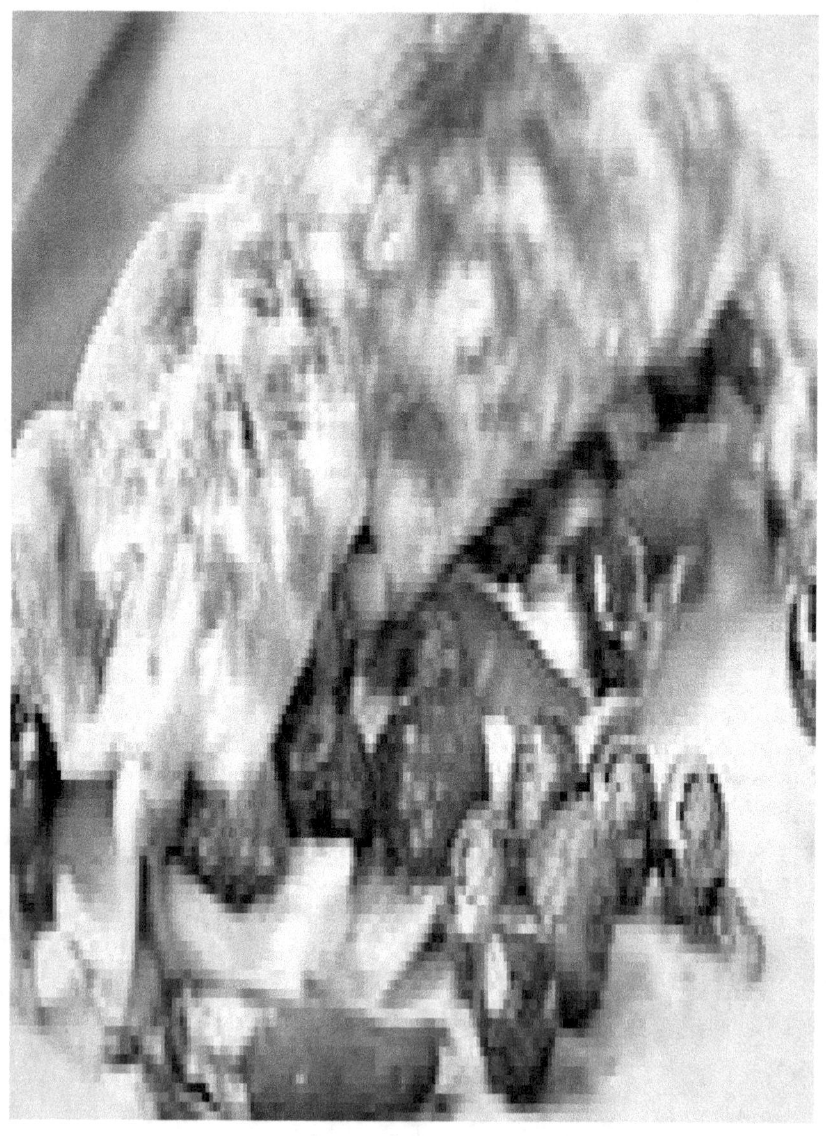

 Prep time= 5 minutes

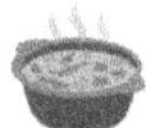 Cooking time= 2 minutes

INGREDIENTS

One big egg
1 tablespoon skim milk
3 cinnamon pinches
100g cottage cheese, 1/2 tsp
rapeseed oil
strawberries, blueberries,
and raspberries, weighing
175g

Nutrient Unit

Kcal: 264
Fat: 12g
Saturates 3.9g
Carbs: 18.9g
Sugars: 15g
Fiber: 4g
Protein: 20.5g
low in salt: 1.0g

INSTRUCTION

STEP 1

With milk and cinnamon,
beat an egg. Pour the egg
mixture into a heated 20 cm
non-stick frying pan,
swirling to coat the bottom
evenly. Cook till the bottom
is golden and set for a few
minutes. You don't have to
turn it over.

STEP 2

Place spread cheese over,
and top with berries on a
platter. Wrap up and dish
out.

Sausages with oregano, mushrooms and olives

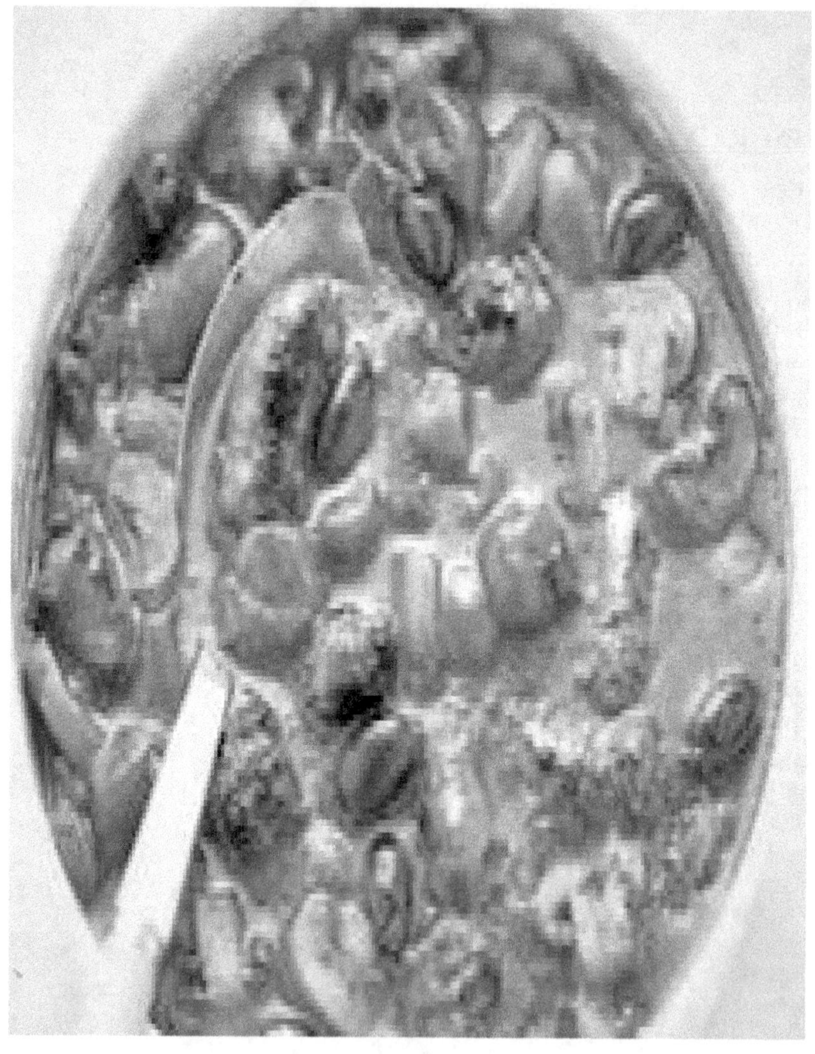

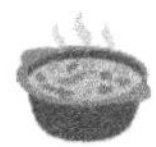 Prep time= 10 minutes

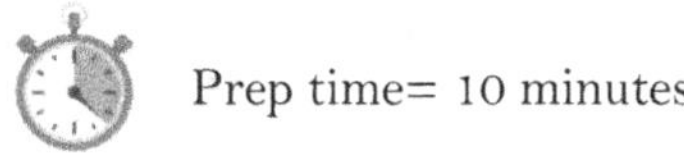 Cooking time= 20 minutes

INGREDIENTS

50-gram package of low-fat
sausage
Sunflower oil, 1 teaspoon
1 teaspoon dried oregano
2 chopped garlic cloves
400g can be cherry tomatoes
or chopped.
200 ml beef broth
Black olives in brine, 100g,
pitted
500g of thickly sliced
mushrooms

Nutrient Unit

Kcal: 263
Fat: 11.9g
Saturates 15.9g
Carbs: 12.2g
Sugars: 3.5g
Fiber: 4.9g
Protein: 20g
low in salt: 1.93g

INSTRUCTION

STEP 1

Cut the sausages into
meatball-sized pieces using
kitchen shears. The pieces
should be fried in hot oil for
about 5 minutes, or until
golden all over.

STEP 2

After one additional minute,
add the oregano, garlic,
tomatoes, stock, olives, and
mushrooms.

STEP 3

Simmer for 15 minutes, or
until the sauce has slightly
reduced and the sausages are
thoroughly cooked. Serve
with spaghetti or mashed
potatoes.

Spiced carrot and lentil soup

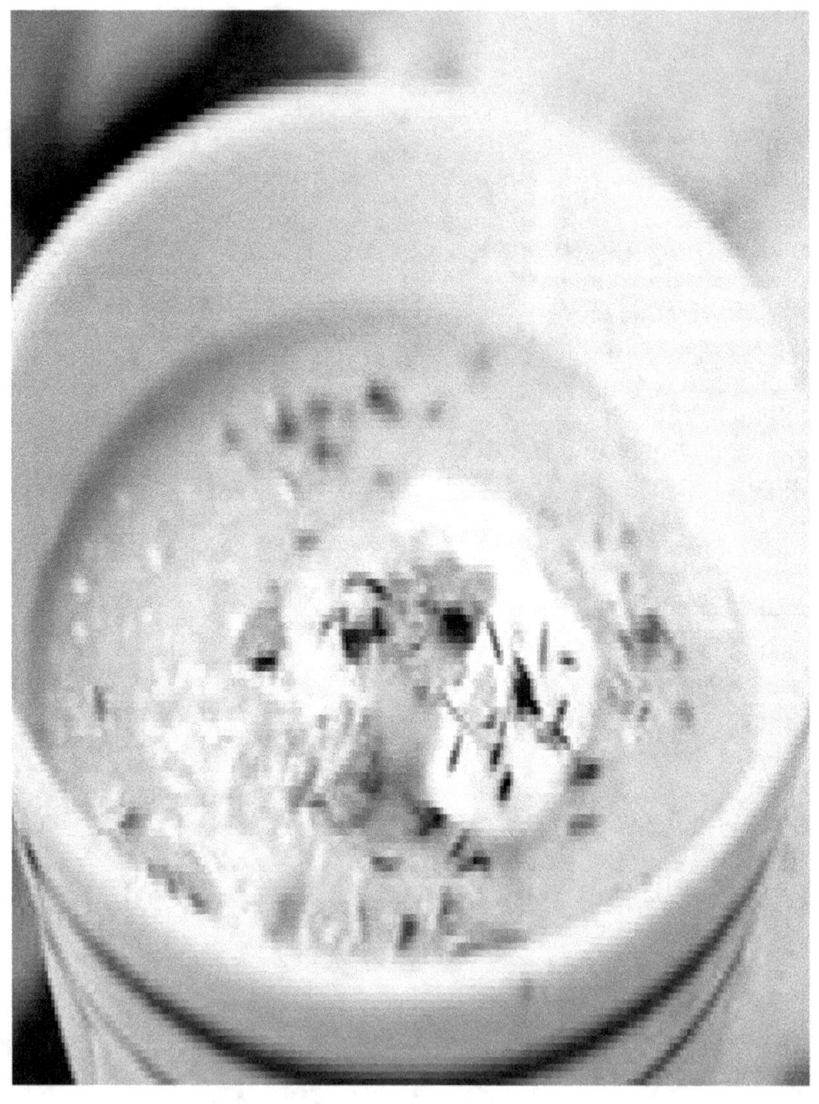

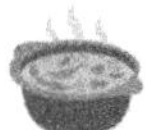 Prep time= 10 minutes

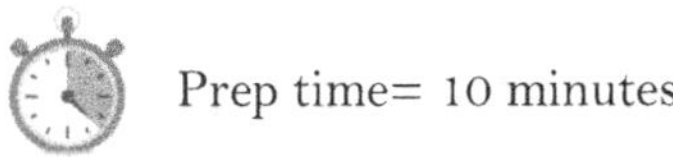 Cooking time= 15 minutes

INGREDIENTS

Cumin seeds, 2 teaspoons, and a dash of red pepper flakes

2 tablespoons of extra virgin olive oil

No need to peel 600 grams of rinsed and coarsely chopped carrots.

140 grams of split red lentils

1 cup of heated vegetable stock (from a cube is fine)

125ml milk (to make it dairy-free, see "try" below)

To serve: naan bread and simple yogurt

INSTRUCTION

STEP 1

Two tablespoons of cumin seeds and a pinch of red pepper flakes should be dry-fried in a big saucepan over high heat for one minute, or until they begin to jump around the pan and exude their scents.

STEP 2

With a spoon, remove roughly half of the mixture and set it aside. 2 tbsp of olive oil, 600 grams of coarsely chopped carrots, 140 grams of split red lentils, 1 liter of hot vegetable stock, and 125 milliliters of milk are added to the pan and heated to boiling.

Nutrient Unit

Kcal: 238
Fat: 6.9g
Saturates 1g
Carbs: 33.9g
Sugars: 0g
Fiber: 4.9g
Protein: 11g
low in salt: 0.24g

INSTRUCTION

STEP 3

Lentils should be simmered for 15 minutes or until they have enlarged and softened.

Smooth up the soup with a stick blender or a food processor, or leave it chunky if you want.

STEP 4

Add salt and pepper to taste, followed by a dollop of plain yogurt and a sprinkle of the saved toasted spices. Serve with warm naan flatbread.

Lifestyle Practices for Brain Health

Regular Physical Activity: Exercise regularly, such as brisk walking, jogging, swimming, or yoga, helps to improve blood flow to the brain. As a result, the transport of vital nutrients and oxygen is enhanced, maintaining brain health and lowering the risk of cognitive decline.

Balanced Diet: A balanced diet that includes whole grains, lean proteins, healthy fats, and a range of fruits and vegetables that provide the nutrients needed for brain function. Omega-3 fatty acids, which are excellent for the brain, are found in salmon and other fatty fish.

Mental Stimulation: Keep your mind busy by partaking in mental exercises. Maintaining cognitive flexibility and memory can be facilitated by reading, solving puzzles, picking up a new skill, or taking part in intellectual dialogues.

Obtain 7-9 hours of sound sleep: every night as a top priority. Memory consolidation, emotion processing, and supporting general brain function all depend on sleep.

Social Engagement: Social interaction is crucial for maintaining brain health. Feelings of isolation can be avoided and cognitive performance can be stimulated by social interaction with friends, family, and other people.

Water: Adequate water helps the brain's ability to receive oxygen and nutrients. Make an effort to consume enough water throughout the day.

Limit Alcohol and Tobacco Use: Both excessive alcohol use and tobacco use raise the risk of cognitive deterioration. To safeguard your brain's health, limit or avoid certain chemicals.

Routine Medical Exams: Regular medical exams enable the early detection and control of health disorders like high blood pressure, diabetes, or high cholesterol that may have an impact on your brain's health.

Stay Mentally Active: Take up a new pastime or study a new language to keep your mind active. You can also play strategy games or acquire a new skill. These actions strengthen cognitive resilience by stimulating neuronal connections.

Hydration and Its Impact on Cognition

Water is a fundamental component of the human body, and its role extends beyond basic physiological processes. Research has shown that even mild dehydration can lead to cognitive impairments, affecting attention, memory, and overall cognitive performance. Dehydration can lead to reduced blood volume and blood flow to the brain, which in turn can compromise oxygen and nutrient delivery to brain cells. This can result in decreased cognitive processing speed, difficulty concentrating, and impaired short-term memory.

It's recommended that adults aim for around 8 glasses (about 2 liters) of water per day, although individual hydration needs can vary based on factors such as age, activity level, and climate. Monitoring urine color is a practical way to gauge hydration status; pale yellow urine is generally indicative of adequate hydration.

For individuals who may struggle to maintain proper hydration, especially older adults who might have a blunted thirst sensation, it's essential to establish a regular hydration routine. Incorporating water-rich foods, such as fruits and vegetables, can also contribute to overall hydration levels.

Water is an integral component of our body's overall function, and the brain is no exception. Approximately 75% of the human brain is composed of water, highlighting its crucial role in supporting various cognitive processes. Here are some key ways in which water influences brain function:

1. Cellular Communication: Adequate hydration ensures efficient neurotransmitter production and transport, facilitating communication between brain cells. This is vital for memory, learning, and overall cognitive function.

2. Nutrient Transport: Water carries essential nutrients and oxygen to brain cells, promoting their proper function and supporting energy metabolism. Proper hydration ensures a steady supply of these vital elements.

3. Waste Removal: The brain generates metabolic waste that needs to be efficiently removed. Water helps in flushing out these waste products, preventing their accumulation and potential cognitive impairment.

4. Temperature Regulation: The brain is sensitive to changes in temperature, and water helps regulate body temperature. Maintaining proper hydration helps prevent overheating, which can negatively impact cognitive abilities.

5. Electrolyte Balance: Electrolytes, such as sodium and potassium, play a crucial role in transmitting electrical signals within the brain. Proper hydration maintains the balance of these electrolytes, supporting smooth nerve signaling.

6. Cerebrospinal Fluid: Water is a primary component of cerebrospinal fluid, which cushions the brain and spinal cord from physical impact. Hydration helps maintain the optimal volume and composition of this fluid.

CHAPTER SIX

Herbal Infusions for Cognitive Wellness

Herbal infusions, derived from various plants, have gained attention for their potential cognitive-enhancing properties. These natural compounds are rich in antioxidants, polyphenols, and other bioactive compounds that may contribute to brain health. Here are a few herbal infusions that have shown promise in supporting cognitive wellness.

Ginkgo Biloba: Extracted from the leaves of the Ginkgo tree, this infusion has been associated with improved blood circulation to the brain. It contains flavonoids and terpenoids that might aid memory and cognitive function.

Rosemary: Known for its aromatic properties, rosemary infusion contains rosmarinic acid, which has been linked to cognitive enhancement. It may potentially improve focus and alertness.

Turmeric: The active compound in turmeric, curcumin, has potent anti-inflammatory and antioxidant effects. Regular consumption of turmeric infusion might help protect brain cells and support cognitive function.

Peppermint: This refreshing infusion is known to invigorate the senses. Its menthol content could aid in reducing mental fatigue and improving concentration.

Bacopa Monnieri: Derived from a traditional Ayurvedic herb, bacopa infusion is believed to have neuroprotective properties. It may positively impact memory and cognitive performance.

Gotu Kola: Gotu kola has been traditionally used to support brain health. It is thought to promote healthy circulation and provide a calming effect, which may aid in reducing stress-related cognitive decline.

Lemon Balm: Lemon balm is known for its calming properties and potential to reduce anxiety. By alleviating stress, it indirectly supports cognitive function.

Physical Activity and Brain Vitality

Consistent physical activity has been shown via considerable research to have a significant impact on brain health. Numerous facets of brain health, including cognitive function, emotional control, and the avoidance of neurodegenerative diseases, are positively impacted by regular exercise you need to consider these key points:

1. Enhanced Cognitive Function: Exercise encourages better blood circulation, which improves the supply of oxygen and nutrients to brain cells. The growth of new neurons and the development of brain connections are supported by this increased blood flow, which improves cognitive function, memory retention, and learning capacity.

2. Balance of Neurotransmitters: Exercise triggers the release of neurotransmitters like dopamine, serotonin, and endorphins. These substances are essential for controlling mood, reducing stress, and maintaining general mental health.

3. Neuroplasticity: The brain's capacity to modify and rearrange itself in response to experiences is influenced by physical activity. For learning, injury rehabilitation, and preserving cognitive function as we age, this plasticity is essential.

4. Decreased Risk of Neurodegenerative Disorders: Alzheimer's and Parkinson's illnesses are less common in people who engage in regular physical activity. Delaying the beginning of cognitive decline, aids in the preservation of brain volume and structure.

5. Stress Reduction: Exercise helps to lower stress and anxiety levels by encouraging the release of hormones that reduce tension and foster relaxation. The general mental clarity and attention are enhanced as a result.

6. Sleep Enhancement: It has been demonstrated that exercise enhances the quality of sleep, which is crucial for maintaining brain health. The development of memory and cognitive functions is supported by adequate sleep.

According to your physical capabilities and preferences, incorporating a balanced exercise program into your daily routine will considerably improve the health of your brain. I advise speaking with a fitness expert before beginning any new training regimen to ensure a safe and suitable schedule.

Exercise's Influence on Brain Plasticity

Brain plasticity, also known as neuroplasticity, refers to the brain's remarkable ability to reorganize its structure, function, and connections in response to experiences and environmental changes. Recent research highlights the profound impact of regular exercise on enhancing brain plasticity, leading to improved cognitive function and overall brain health.

Exercise and Brain-Derived Neurotrophic Factor (BDNF)

Exercise has been shown to stimulate the release of Brain-Derived Neurotrophic Factor (BDNF), a protein crucial for promoting neuronal growth, survival, and synaptic plasticity. Increased BDNF levels are associated with enhanced synaptic connections and improved learning and memory.

Neurogenesis: Physical activity, particularly aerobic exercises such as running or swimming, has been linked to increased neurogenesis – the formation of new neurons in the hippocampus, a region vital for learning and memory. Neurogenesis contributes to the brain's ability to adapt to new information and experiences.

Synaptic Plasticity: Regular exercise fosters synaptic plasticity, the strengthening or weakening of synaptic connections between neurons. This mechanism underlies learning processes and memory consolidation. Exercise-induced synaptic plasticity enhances information processing and adaptability of the brain.

Cerebral Blood Flow and Oxygenation: Exercise enhances cerebral blood flow and oxygen delivery to the brain. Improved blood flow ensures the delivery of essential nutrients and oxygen required for optimal neuronal function. This increase in blood flow supports the brain's ability to adapt to new challenges.

Neuroprotective Effects: Exercise plays a pivotal role in maintaining brain health by reducing oxidative stress and inflammation. These neuroprotective effects contribute to preserving existing neurons and their connections, preventing cognitive decline associated with aging.

Clinical Implications: Understanding the impact of exercise on brain plasticity has important clinical implications. Incorporating regular physical activity into one's routine can aid in mitigating cognitive decline associated with aging, reducing the risk of neurodegenerative diseases, and enhancing overall cognitive function. Furthermore, exercise can be prescribed as an adjunctive therapy in various neurological and psychiatric conditions to support cognitive rehabilitation.

CHAPTER SEVEN

Creating a Brain-Healthy Workout Routine

Maintaining a healthy body goes hand in hand with preserving cognitive function and promoting brain health. Just as regular exercise is essential for your physical well-being, it also plays a vital role in nurturing your cognitive abilities and guarding against neurological decline. In this note, we will explore the key principles of crafting a brain-healthy workout routine.

Aerobic Exercise: Incorporating regular aerobic exercise into your routine is paramount. Activities such as brisk walking, jogging, swimming, and cycling increase blood flow to the brain, delivering oxygen and vital nutrients. Aim for 150 or more minutes per week of aerobic activity at a moderate level.

Strength Training: Building and maintaining muscle mass through strength training exercises are equally crucial. Muscle tissue releases chemicals that promote brain health. At least two days a week should be devoted to strength training with an emphasis on all major muscle groups.

Balance and Coordination: Engage in activities that challenge your balance and coordination, like yoga, tai chi, or dancing. These activities stimulate various parts of the brain responsible for motor skills and spatial awareness.

Mind-Body Connection: Mindfulness exercises, such as meditation, can reduce stress and improve concentration. Regular practice can enhance brain plasticity, making it easier for your brain to adapt and learn new things.

Variety: Rotate your workouts to engage different muscle groups and cognitive functions. Cross-training not only prevents boredom but also maximizes brain benefits by exposing it to diverse challenges.

Adequate Rest: Allow your body and brain to recover. For the brain to work properly and consolidate memories, one needs quality sleep. Aim for seven to nine hours of unbroken sleep each night.

Nutrition: A brain-healthy diet complements your exercise routine. Consume a diet that is well-balanced and full of fresh produce, whole grains, lean protein, and healthy fats. Omega-3 fatty acids, found in fatty fish like salmon, have been linked to improved brain health.

Social Interaction: Incorporate activities that involve social interaction, like group workouts or team sports. Social engagement can enhance cognitive resilience.

Consult a Professional: If you have specific health concerns or medical conditions, consult with a healthcare provider or fitness expert to tailor your exercise routine to your needs and abilities.

CONCLUSION

The Brain Diet Recipes offer a holistic approach to nourishing both body and mind in the golden years of life. Through this culinary journey, we have explored the power of nutrient-rich ingredients, carefully selected to promote cognitive health and overall well-being. The recipes featured here prioritize foods that are rich in antioxidants, omega-3 fatty acids, vitamins, and minerals, all of which play a vital role in maintaining brain health.

We've discovered that simple dietary changes can have a profound impact on memory, focus, and cognitive function. The incorporation of colorful fruits and vegetables, whole grains, lean proteins, and healthy fats into your daily meals can help protect against cognitive decline, reduce the risk of age-related diseases, and enhance your quality of life.

It's important to keep in mind consistency as you start your Brain Diet journey. Gradually incorporating these recipes into your daily routine can lead to long-lasting positive effects on your brain health. Moreover, staying hydrated and maintaining a healthy lifestyle, including regular physical activity and adequate sleep, will complement the benefits of this diet.

In this ever-advancing world, where the demands on our cognitive abilities are constantly increasing, it's crucial to invest in the health of our brains. By adopting and adapting the Brain Diet Recipes for Seniors, you are taking a proactive step towards preserving your cognitive vitality. Remember, your brain is a precious asset that deserves the best care possible.

Each delicious meal from this collection, let it serves as a reminder of the importance of nourishing your brain. Embrace this diet not as a chore, but as a celebration of the incredible machine that is your brain. Your cognitive health is worth every effort, and by following these recipes, you are investing in a brighter, sharper, and more fulfilling future.

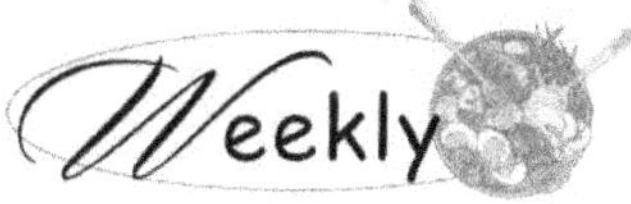

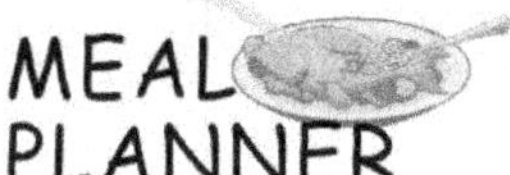

WEEK _______________________   MONTH _______________________

MONDAY

BREAKFAST:

LUNCH:

DINNER:

TUESDAY

BREAKFAST:

LUNCH:

DINNER:

WEDNESDAY

BREAKFAST:

LUNCH:

DINNER:

THURSDAY

BREAKFAST:

LUNCH:

DINNER:

FRIDAY

BREAKFAST:

LUNCH:

DINNER:

SATURDAY

BREAKFAST:

LUNCH:

DINNER:

SUNDAY

BREAKFAST:

LUNCH:

DINNER:

INGREDIENT LIST

- _______________________
- _______________________
- _______________________
- _______________________
- _______________________
- _______________________
- _______________________
- _______________________
- _______________________
- _______________________
- _______________________

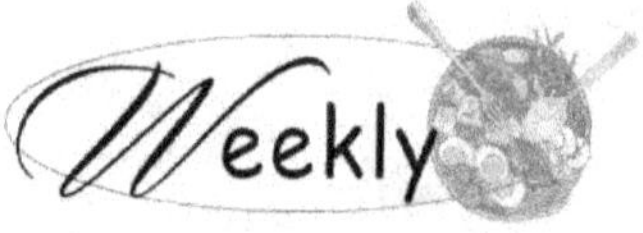

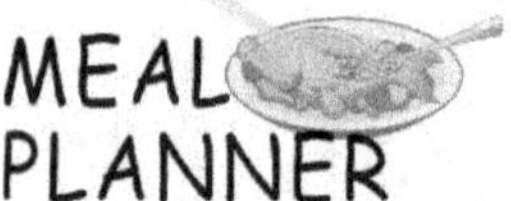

WEEK ___________________   MONTH ___________________

MONDAY
BREAKFAST:
LUNCH:
DINNER:

TUESDAY
BREAKFAST:
LUNCH:
DINNER:

WEDNESDAY
BREAKFAST:
LUNCH:
DINNER:

THURSDAY
BREAKFAST:
LUNCH:
DINNER:

FRIDAY
BREAKFAST:
LUNCH:
DINNER:

SATURDAY
BREAKFAST:
LUNCH:
DINNER:

SUNDAY
BREAKFAST:
LUNCH:
DINNER:

INGREDIENT LIST
◇ ___________________
◇ ___________________
◇ ___________________
◇ ___________________
◇ ___________________
◇ ___________________
◇ ___________________
◇ ___________________
◇ ___________________
◇ ___________________
◇ ___________________
◇ ___________________

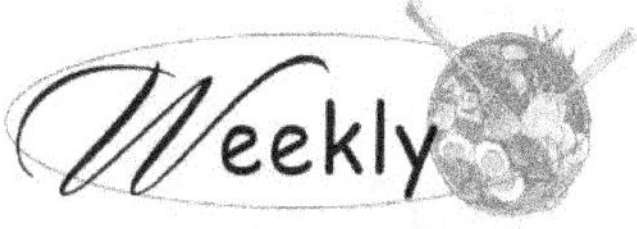

Weekly MEAL PLANNER

WEEK ___________________   **MONTH** ___________________

MONDAY

BREAKFAST:

LUNCH:

DINNER:

TUESDAY

BREAKFAST:

LUNCH:

DINNER:

WEDNESDAY

BREAKFAST:

LUNCH:

DINNER:

THURSDAY

BREAKFAST:

LUNCH:

DINNER:

FRIDAY

BREAKFAST:

LUNCH:

DINNER:

SATURDAY

BREAKFAST:

LUNCH:

DINNER:

SUNDAY

BREAKFAST:

LUNCH:

DINNER:

INGREDIENT LIST

✧ ___________________________

✧ ___________________________

✧ ___________________________

✧ ___________________________

✧ ___________________________

✧ ___________________________

✧ ___________________________

✧ ___________________________

✧ ___________________________

✧ ___________________________

✧ ___________________________

✧ ___________________________

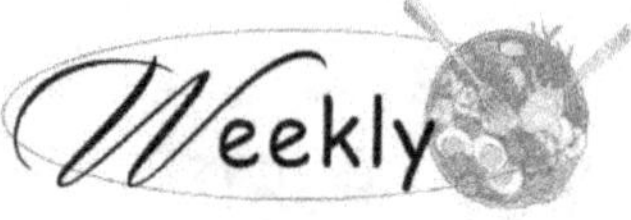

Weekly MEAL PLANNER

WEEK _______________________   MONTH _______________________

MONDAY
BREAKFAST;
LUNCH;
DINNER;

TUESDAY
BREAKFAST;
LUNCH;
DINNER;

WEDNESDAY
BREAKFAST;
LUNCH;
DINNER;

THURSDAY
BREAKFAST;
LUNCH;
DINNER;

FRIDAY
BREAKFAST;
LUNCH;
DINNER;

SATURDAY
BREAKFAST;
LUNCH;
DINNER;

SUNDAY
BREAKFAST;
LUNCH;
DINNER;

INGREDIENT LIST
✧ _______________________
✧ _______________________
✧ _______________________
✧ _______________________
✧ _______________________
✧ _______________________
✧ _______________________
✧ _______________________
✧ _______________________
✧ _______________________
✧ _______________________

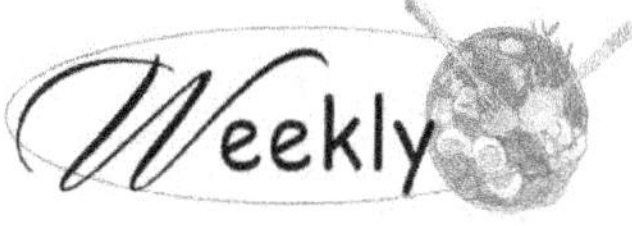 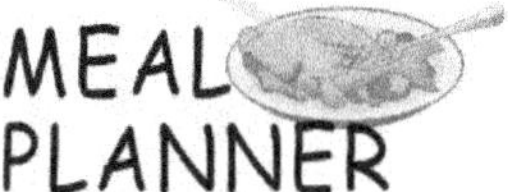

Weekly MEAL PLANNER

WEEK _______________________   MONTH _______________________

MONDAY

BREAKFAST:

LUNCH:

DINNER:

TUESDAY

BREAKFAST:

LUNCH:

DINNER:

WEDNESDAY

BREAKFAST:

LUNCH:

DINNER:

THURSDAY

BREAKFAST:

LUNCH:

DINNER:

FRIDAY

BREAKFAST:

LUNCH:

DINNER:

SATURDAY

BREAKFAST:

LUNCH:

DINNER:

SUNDAY

BREAKFAST:

LUNCH:

DINNER:

INGREDIENT LIST

◇ _______________________
◇ _______________________
◇ _______________________
◇ _______________________
◇ _______________________
◇ _______________________
◇ _______________________
◇ _______________________
◇ _______________________
◇ _______________________
◇ _______________________
◇ _______________________

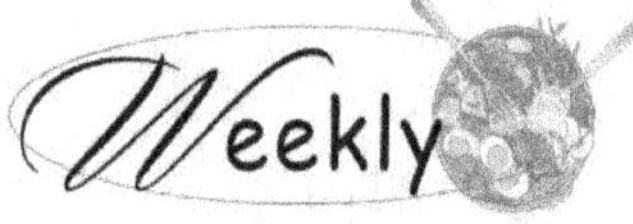

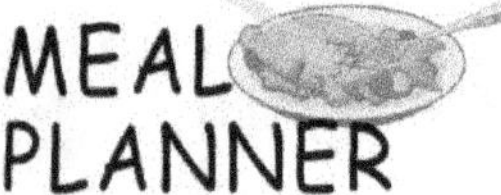

WEEK _______________   MONTH _______________

MONDAY

BREAKFAST:

LUNCH:

DINNER:

TUESDAY

BREAKFAST:

LUNCH:

DINNER:

WEDNESDAY

BREAKFAST:

LUNCH:

DINNER:

THURSDAY

BREAKFAST:

LUNCH:

DINNER:

FRIDAY

BREAKFAST:

LUNCH:

DINNER:

SATURDAY

BREAKFAST:

LUNCH:

DINNER:

SUNDAY

BREAKFAST:

LUNCH:

DINNER:

INGREDIENT LIST

◇ _______________
◇ _______________
◇ _______________
◇ _______________
◇ _______________
◇ _______________
◇ _______________
◇ _______________
◇ _______________
◇ _______________
◇ _______________
◇ _______________

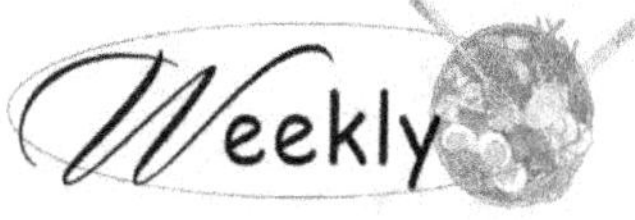

MEAL PLANNER

WEEK _______________   **MONTH** _______________

MONDAY

BREAKFAST:

LUNCH:

DINNER:

TUESDAY

BREAKFAST:

LUNCH:

DINNER:

WEDNESDAY

BREAKFAST:

LUNCH:

DINNER:

THURSDAY

BREAKFAST:

LUNCH:

DINNER:

FRIDAY

BREAKFAST:

LUNCH:

DINNER:

SATURDAY

BREAKFAST:

LUNCH:

DINNER:

SUNDAY

BREAKFAST:

LUNCH:

DINNER:

INGREDIENT LIST

◇ _______________
◇ _______________
◇ _______________
◇ _______________
◇ _______________
◇ _______________
◇ _______________
◇ _______________
◇ _______________
◇ _______________
◇ _______________
◇ _______________

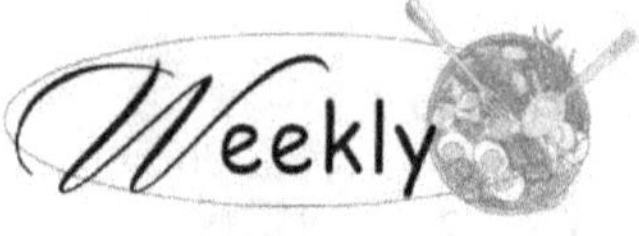 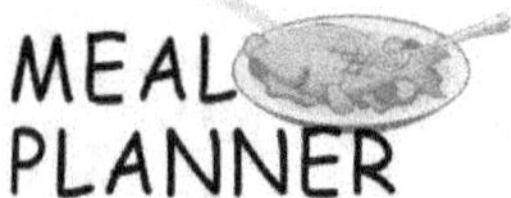

Weekly MEAL PLANNER

WEEK _____________________   MONTH _____________________

MONDAY

BREAKFAST:

LUNCH:

DINNER:

TUESDAY

BREAKFAST:

LUNCH:

DINNER:

WEDNESDAY

BREAKFAST:

LUNCH:

DINNER:

THURSDAY

BREAKFAST:

LUNCH:

DINNER:

FRIDAY

BREAKFAST:

LUNCH:

DINNER:

SATURDAY

BREAKFAST:

LUNCH:

DINNER:

SUNDAY

BREAKFAST:

LUNCH:

DINNER:

INGREDIENT LIST

◇ _____________________

◇ _____________________

◇ _____________________

◇ _____________________

◇ _____________________

◇ _____________________

◇ _____________________

◇ _____________________

◇ _____________________

◇ _____________________

◇ _____________________

◇ _____________________

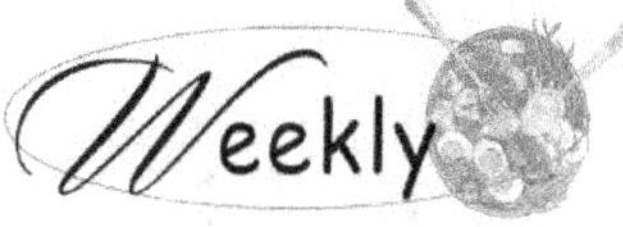 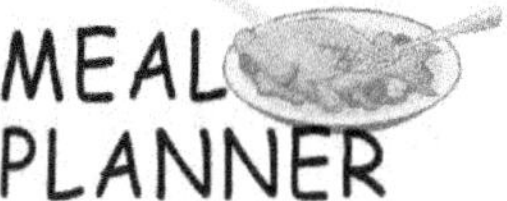

Weekly MEAL PLANNER

WEEK _______________   MONTH _______________

MONDAY

BREAKFAST:

LUNCH:

DINNER:

TUESDAY

BREAKFAST:

LUNCH:

DINNER:

WEDNESDAY

BREAKFAST:

LUNCH:

DINNER:

THURSDAY

BREAKFAST:

LUNCH:

DINNER:

FRIDAY

BREAKFAST:

LUNCH:

DINNER:

SATURDAY

BREAKFAST:

LUNCH:

DINNER:

SUNDAY

BREAKFAST:

LUNCH:

DINNER:

INGREDIENT LIST

- ◇ _______________
- ◇ _______________
- ◇ _______________
- ◇ _______________
- ◇ _______________
- ◇ _______________
- ◇ _______________
- ◇ _______________
- ◇ _______________
- ◇ _______________
- ◇ _______________
- ◇ _______________

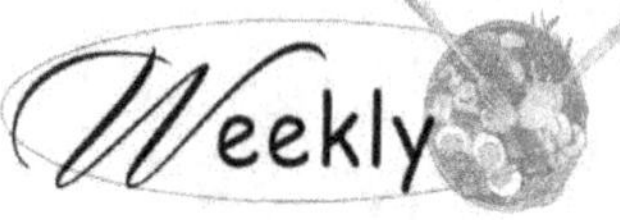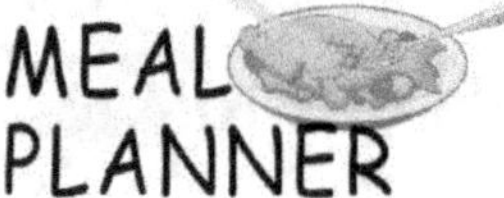

Weekly MEAL PLANNER

WEEK _______________________   **MONTH** _______________________

MONDAY

BREAKFAST:

LUNCH:

DINNER:

TUESDAY

BREAKFAST:

LUNCH:

DINNER:

WEDNESDAY

BREAKFAST:

LUNCH:

DINNER:

THURSDAY

BREAKFAST:

LUNCH:

DINNER:

FRIDAY

BREAKFAST:

LUNCH:

DINNER:

SATURDAY

BREAKFAST:

LUNCH:

DINNER:

SUNDAY

BREAKFAST:

LUNCH:

DINNER:

INGREDIENT LIST

- ◇ _______________________
- ◇ _______________________
- ◇ _______________________
- ◇ _______________________
- ◇ _______________________
- ◇ _______________________
- ◇ _______________________
- ◇ _______________________
- ◇ _______________________
- ◇ _______________________
- ◇ _______________________
- ◇ _______________________
- ◇ _______________________

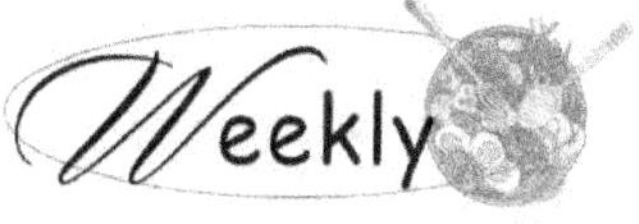 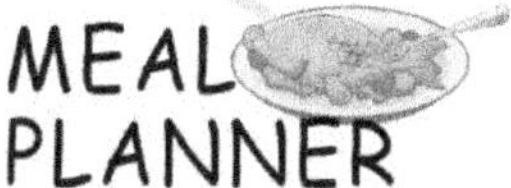

Weekly MEAL PLANNER

WEEK _______________   **MONTH** _______________

MONDAY

BREAKFAST;

LUNCH;

DINNER;

TUESDAY

BREAKFAST;

LUNCH;

DINNER;

WEDNESDAY

BREAKFAST;

LUNCH;

DINNER;

THURSDAY

BREAKFAST;

LUNCH;

DINNER;

FRIDAY

BREAKFAST;

LUNCH;

DINNER;

SATURDAY

BREAKFAST:

LUNCH;

DINNER;

SUNDAY

BREAKFAST;

LUNCH;

DINNER;

INGREDIENT LIST

◇ _______________
◇ _______________
◇ _______________
◇ _______________
◇ _______________
◇ _______________
◇ _______________
◇ _______________
◇ _______________
◇ _______________
◇ _______________
◇ _______________

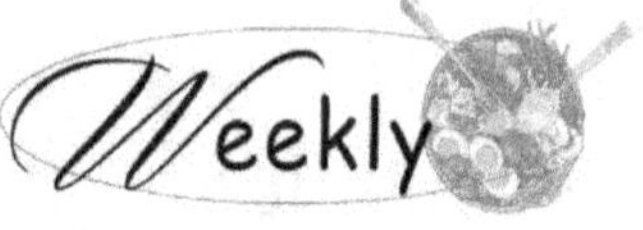
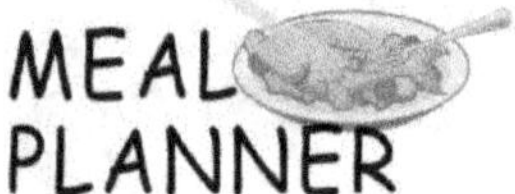

Weekly MEAL PLANNER

WEEK _______________________   MONTH _______________________

MONDAY

BREAKFAST:

LUNCH:

DINNER:

TUESDAY

BREAKFAST:

LUNCH:

DINNER:

WEDNESDAY

BREAKFAST:

LUNCH:

DINNER:

THURSDAY

BREAKFAST:

LUNCH:

DINNER:

FRIDAY

BREAKFAST:

LUNCH:

DINNER:

SATURDAY

BREAKFAST:

LUNCH:

DINNER:

SUNDAY

BREAKFAST:

LUNCH:

DINNER:

INGREDIENT LIST

- ✧ _______________________
- ✧ _______________________
- ✧ _______________________
- ✧ _______________________
- ✧ _______________________
- ✧ _______________________
- ✧ _______________________
- ✧ _______________________
- ✧ _______________________
- ✧ _______________________
- ✧ _______________________
- ✧ _______________________

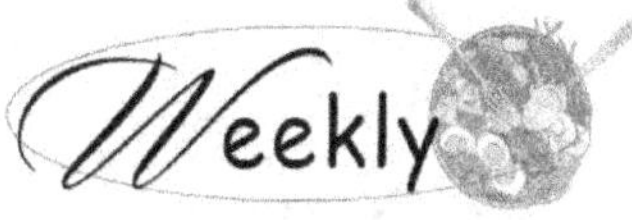

Weekly MEAL PLANNER

WEEK __________________   **MONTH** __________________

MONDAY

BREAKFAST:

LUNCH:

DINNER:

TUESDAY

BREAKFAST:

LUNCH:

DINNER:

WEDNESDAY

BREAKFAST:

LUNCH:

DINNER:

THURSDAY

BREAKFAST:

LUNCH:

DINNER:

FRIDAY

BREAKFAST:

LUNCH:

DINNER:

SATURDAY

BREAKFAST:

LUNCH:

DINNER:

SUNDAY

BREAKFAST:

LUNCH:

DINNER:

INGREDIENT LIST

◇ __________________
◇ __________________
◇ __________________
◇ __________________
◇ __________________
◇ __________________
◇ __________________
◇ __________________
◇ __________________
◇ __________________
◇ __________________
◇ __________________
◇ __________________

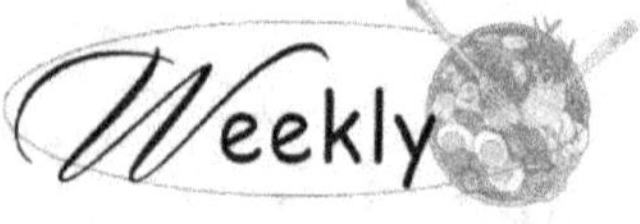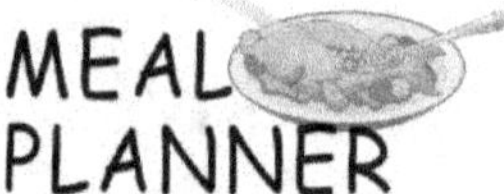

Weekly MEAL PLANNER

WEEK _______________________   **MONTH** _______________________

MONDAY

BREAKFAST:
LUNCH:
DINNER:

TUESDAY

BREAKFAST:
LUNCH:
DINNER:

WEDNESDAY

BREAKFAST:
LUNCH:
DINNER:

THURSDAY

BREAKFAST:
LUNCH:
DINNER:

FRIDAY

BREAKFAST:
LUNCH:
DINNER:

SATURDAY

BREAKFAST:
LUNCH:
DINNER:

SUNDAY

BREAKFAST:
LUNCH:
DINNER:

INGREDIENT LIST

◇ _______________________
◇ _______________________
◇ _______________________
◇ _______________________
◇ _______________________
◇ _______________________
◇ _______________________
◇ _______________________
◇ _______________________
◇ _______________________
◇ _______________________
◇ _______________________

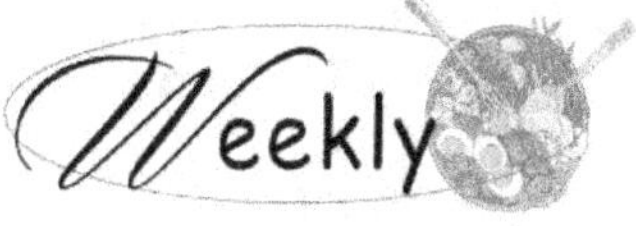 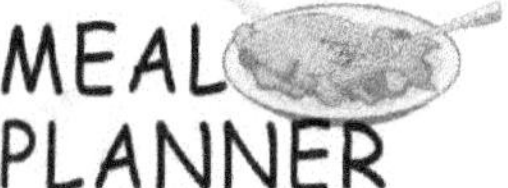

Weekly MEAL PLANNER

WEEK ______________________   MONTH ______________________

MONDAY

BREAKFAST:

LUNCH:

DINNER:

TUESDAY

BREAKFAST:

LUNCH:

DINNER:

WEDNESDAY

BREAKFAST:

LUNCH:

DINNER:

THURSDAY

BREAKFAST:

LUNCH:

DINNER:

FRIDAY

BREAKFAST:

LUNCH:

DINNER:

SATURDAY

BREAKFAST:

LUNCH:

DINNER:

SUNDAY

BREAKFAST:

LUNCH:

DINNER:

INGREDIENT LIST

◇ ______________________
◇ ______________________
◇ ______________________
◇ ______________________
◇ ______________________
◇ ______________________
◇ ______________________
◇ ______________________
◇ ______________________
◇ ______________________
◇ ______________________
◇ ______________________

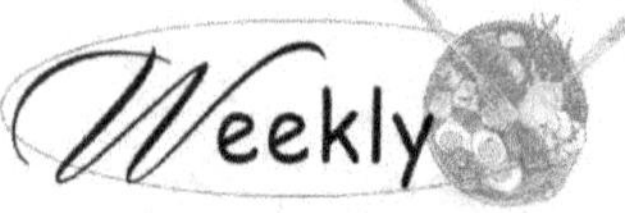 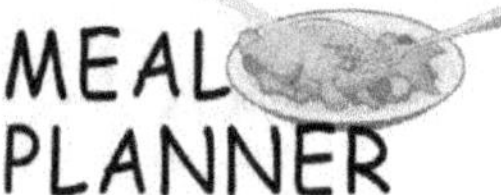

Weekly MEAL PLANNER

WEEK _______________________   **MONTH** _______________________

MONDAY

BREAKFAST:

LUNCH:

DINNER:

TUESDAY

BREAKFAST:

LUNCH:

DINNER:

WEDNESDAY

BREAKFAST:

LUNCH:

DINNER:

THURSDAY

BREAKFAST:

LUNCH:

DINNER:

FRIDAY

BREAKFAST:

LUNCH:

DINNER:

SATURDAY

BREAKFAST:

LUNCH:

DINNER:

SUNDAY

BREAKFAST:

LUNCH:

DINNER:

INGREDIENT LIST

- _______________________
- _______________________
- _______________________
- _______________________
- _______________________
- _______________________
- _______________________
- _______________________
- _______________________
- _______________________
- _______________________
- _______________________

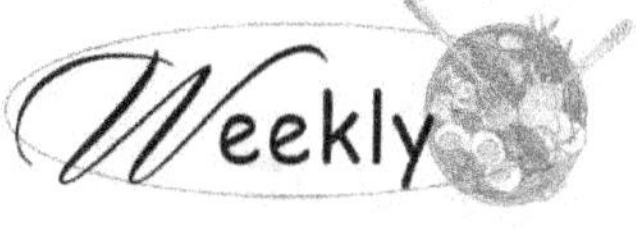

Weekly MEAL PLANNER

WEEK _______________________   MONTH _______________________

MONDAY
BREAKFAST:
LUNCH:
DINNER:

TUESDAY
BREAKFAST:
LUNCH:
DINNER:

WEDNESDAY
BREAKFAST:
LUNCH:
DINNER:

THURSDAY
BREAKFAST:
LUNCH:
DINNER:

FRIDAY
BREAKFAST:
LUNCH:
DINNER:

SATURDAY
BREAKFAST:
LUNCH:
DINNER:

SUNDAY
BREAKFAST:
LUNCH:
DINNER:

INGREDIENT LIST
◇ _______________________
◇ _______________________
◇ _______________________
◇ _______________________
◇ _______________________
◇ _______________________
◇ _______________________
◇ _______________________
◇ _______________________
◇ _______________________
◇ _______________________
◇ _______________________

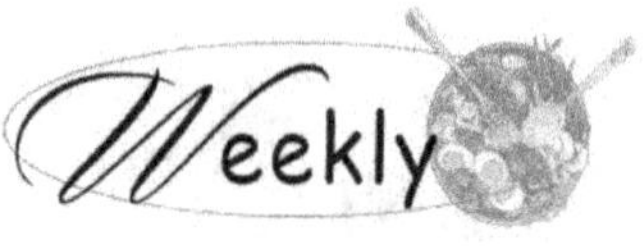

MEAL PLANNER

WEEK _______________________   **MONTH** _______________________

MONDAY

BREAKFAST:

LUNCH:

DINNER:

TUESDAY

BREAKFAST:

LUNCH:

DINNER:

WEDNESDAY

BREAKFAST:

LUNCH:

DINNER:

THURSDAY

BREAKFAST:

LUNCH:

DINNER:

FRIDAY

BREAKFAST:

LUNCH:

DINNER:

SATURDAY

BREAKFAST:

LUNCH:

DINNER:

SUNDAY

BREAKFAST:

LUNCH:

DINNER:

INGREDIENT LIST

◇ _______________________

◇ _______________________

◇ _______________________

◇ _______________________

◇ _______________________

◇ _______________________

◇ _______________________

◇ _______________________

◇ _______________________

◇ _______________________

◇ _______________________

◇ _______________________

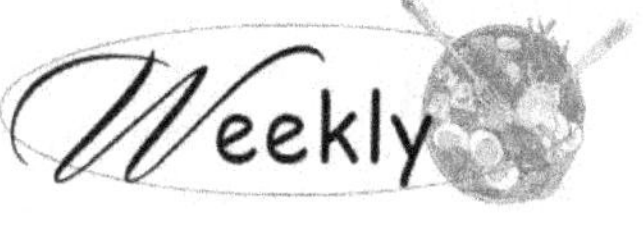

Weekly MEAL PLANNER

WEEK ______________________   **MONTH** ______________________

MONDAY

BREAKFAST;

LUNCH;

DINNER:

TUESDAY

BREAKFAST;

LUNCH;

DINNER;

WEDNESDAY

BREAKFAST;

LUNCH;

DINNER;

THURSDAY

BREAKFAST;

LUNCH;

DINNER;

FRIDAY

BREAKFAST;

LUNCH;

DINNER;

SATURDAY

BREAKFAST;

LUNCH;

DINNER:

SUNDAY

BREAKFAST;

LUNCH;

DINNER;

INGREDIENT LIST

- ______________________
- ______________________
- ______________________
- ______________________
- ______________________
- ______________________
- ______________________
- ______________________
- ______________________
- ______________________
- ______________________
- ______________________

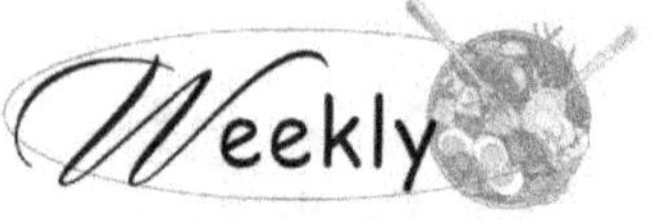 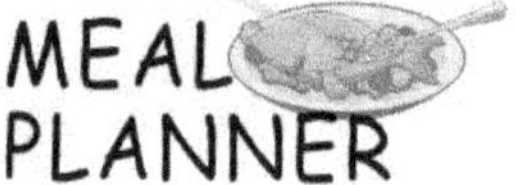

Weekly MEAL PLANNER

WEEK _______________________   MONTH _______________________

MONDAY

BREAKFAST:

LUNCH:

DINNER:

TUESDAY

BREAKFAST:

LUNCH:

DINNER:

WEDNESDAY

BREAKFAST:

LUNCH:

DINNER:

THURSDAY

BREAKFAST:

LUNCH:

DINNER:

FRIDAY

BREAKFAST:

LUNCH:

DINNER:

SATURDAY

BREAKFAST:

LUNCH:

DINNER:

SUNDAY

BREAKFAST:

LUNCH:

DINNER:

INGREDIENT LIST

✧ _______________________

✧ _______________________

✧ _______________________

✧ _______________________

✧ _______________________

✧ _______________________

✧ _______________________

✧ _______________________

✧ _______________________

✧ _______________________

✧ _______________________

✧ _______________________

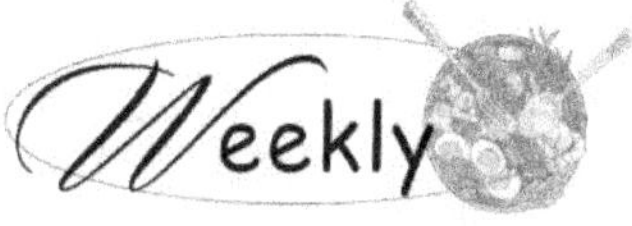 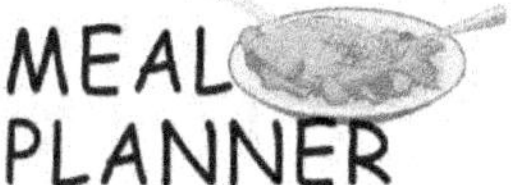

Weekly MEAL PLANNER

WEEK _______________________   MONTH _______________________

MONDAY

BREAKFAST:

LUNCH:

DINNER:

TUESDAY

BREAKFAST:

LUNCH:

DINNER:

WEDNESDAY

BREAKFAST:

LUNCH:

DINNER:

THURSDAY

BREAKFAST:

LUNCH:

DINNER:

FRIDAY

BREAKFAST:

LUNCH,

DINNER:

SATURDAY

BREAKFAST:

LUNCH:

DINNER:

SUNDAY

BREAKFAST:

LUNCH:

DINNER:

INGREDIENT LIST

✧ _______________________
✧ _______________________
✧ _______________________
✧ _______________________
✧ _______________________
✧ _______________________
✧ _______________________
✧ _______________________
✧ _______________________
✧ _______________________
✧ _______________________
✧ _______________________

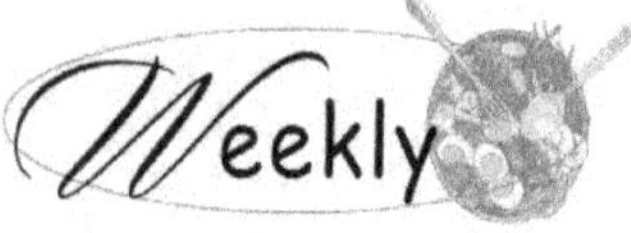 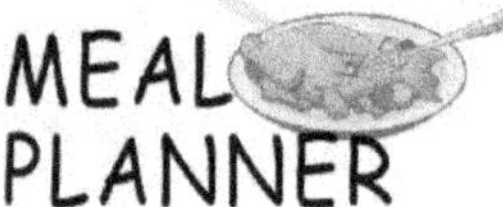

Weekly MEAL PLANNER

WEEK _______________   **MONTH** _______________

MONDAY

BREAKFAST:

LUNCH:

DINNER:

TUESDAY

BREAKFAST:

LUNCH:

DINNER:

WEDNESDAY

BREAKFAST:

LUNCH:

DINNER:

THURSDAY

BREAKFAST:

LUNCH:

DINNER:

FRIDAY

BREAKFAST:

LUNCH:

DINNER:

SATURDAY

BREAKFAST:

LUNCH:

DINNER:

SUNDAY

BREAKFAST:

LUNCH:

DINNER:

INGREDIENT LIST

- ______________________
- ______________________
- ______________________
- ______________________
- ______________________
- ______________________
- ______________________
- ______________________
- ______________________
- ______________________
- ______________________
- ______________________

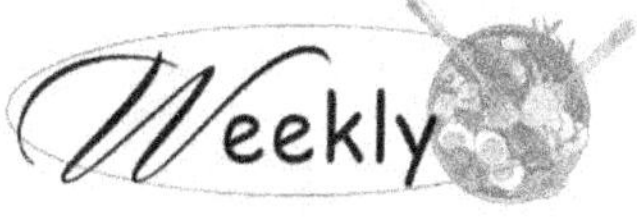

Weekly MEAL PLANNER

WEEK __________________________   MONTH __________________________

MONDAY
BREAKFAST:
LUNCH:
DINNER:

TUESDAY
BREAKFAST:
LUNCH:
DINNER:

WEDNESDAY
BREAKFAST:
LUNCH:
DINNER:

THURSDAY
BREAKFAST:
LUNCH:
DINNER:

FRIDAY
BREAKFAST:
LUNCH:
DINNER:

SATURDAY
BREAKFAST:
LUNCH:
DINNER:

SUNDAY
BREAKFAST:
LUNCH:
DINNER:

INGREDIENT LIST
- ________________________
- ________________________
- ________________________
- ________________________
- ________________________
- ________________________
- ________________________
- ________________________
- ________________________
- ________________________
- ________________________
- ________________________

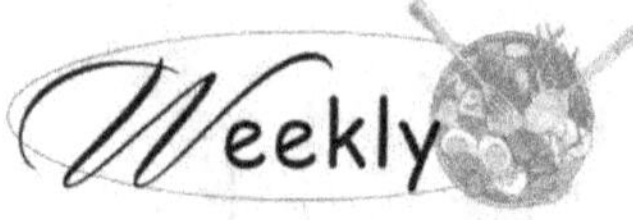
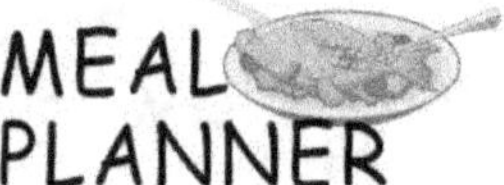

Weekly MEAL PLANNER

WEEK _______________________   **MONTH** _______________________

MONDAY
BREAKFAST:
LUNCH:
DINNER:

TUESDAY
BREAKFAST:
LUNCH:
DINNER:

WEDNESDAY
BREAKFAST:
LUNCH:
DINNER:

THURSDAY
BREAKFAST:
LUNCH:
DINNER:

FRIDAY
BREAKFAST:
LUNCH:
DINNER:

SATURDAY
BREAKFAST:
LUNCH:
DINNER:

SUNDAY
BREAKFAST:
LUNCH:
DINNER:

INGREDIENT LIST

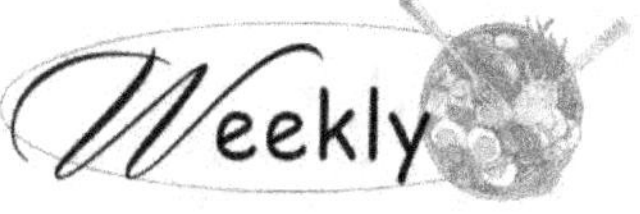

Weekly MEAL PLANNER

WEEK ___________________________   **MONTH** ___________________________

MONDAY

BREAKFAST:

LUNCH:

DINNER:

TUESDAY

BREAKFAST:

LUNCH:

DINNER:

WEDNESDAY

BREAKFAST:

LUNCH:

DINNER:

THURSDAY

BREAKFAST:

LUNCH:

DINNER:

FRIDAY

BREAKFAST:

LUNCH:

DINNER:

SATURDAY

BREAKFAST:

LUNCH:

DINNER:

SUNDAY

BREAKFAST:

LUNCH:

DINNER:

INGREDIENT LIST

✧ ___________________________
✧ ___________________________
✧ ___________________________
✧ ___________________________
✧ ___________________________
✧ ___________________________
✧ ___________________________
✧ ___________________________
✧ ___________________________
✧ ___________________________
✧ ___________________________
✧ ___________________________

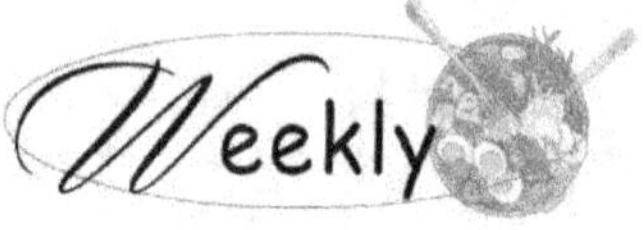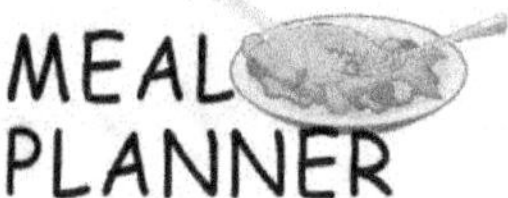

Weekly MEAL PLANNER

WEEK ________________   MONTH ________________

MONDAY

BREAKFAST:

LUNCH:

DINNER:

TUESDAY

BREAKFAST:

LUNCH:

DINNER:

WEDNESDAY

BREAKFAST:

LUNCH:

DINNER:

THURSDAY

BREAKFAST:

LUNCH:

DINNER:

FRIDAY

BREAKFAST:

LUNCH:

DINNER:

SATURDAY

BREAKFAST:

LUNCH:

DINNER:

SUNDAY

BREAKFAST:

LUNCH:

DINNER:

INGREDIENT LIST

◇ ________________

◇ ________________

◇ ________________

◇ ________________

◇ ________________

◇ ________________

◇ ________________

◇ ________________

◇ ________________

◇ ________________

◇ ________________

◇ ________________